Journey to the Finish Line: Surviving Cancer Together

Journey to the Finish Line: Surviving Cancer Together

Van Garner and Virginia Garner

VAN GARNER AND VIRGINIA GARNER
LOS ANGELES, CA

Contents

Contents

Preface

It was the evening of April 12, 2006. Not that I would have known it was evening. I was in a room with lights so bright they pierced my eyelids. I heard a voice. It had to be Virginia. It was always Virginia, my wife of thirty-eight years. I wanted to open my eyes but I couldn't. The doctor interrupted my hazy thoughts: "We have to move you to the bed. It's going to hurt a lot." "Oh no, don't move me," I thought.

As they lifted me, I couldn't stop the scream. The pain penetrated my body from front to back. My eyes opened and I saw my wife, a horrified look on her face. "They have to move you, Van. I know it hurts."

It was no wonder I hurt. An incision ran from my sternum to below my belly button where they had removed a tumor from my jejunum and another ran ten inches across the top of my left hip where they had removed another. The margins around the jejunum tumor were clear, but there was no way to know if the cancer cells were fully removed in the hip because that tumor was too close to the bone.

As I thudded onto the bed, I heard Virginia through my screams, "Van, concentrate on me. I'm going to read to you. We're going to read Dean Karnazes. Do you remember who he is?" I did. Dean Karnazes had just published his book, *Ultramarathon Man*, in which he described his awe-inspiring accomplishments in the world of endurance running. He was in the final planning stages of attempting fifty marathons in fifty states in fifty days.

Since 1997 Virginia had been fighting a deadly form of leukemia. Saved by a miracle drug and feeling strong, she had signed us up for the 2001 Los Angeles Marathon. Not only had we finished L.A., but by the time of my surgery, we had together finished a combined total of forty full and half marathons in addition to surviving three major surgeries, three types of radiation, interferon, Interleukin-2, half a dozen chemotherapy drugs, one experimental drug, scores of CT scans, PET scans, MRIs, and bone marrow biopsies. Having conquered many endurance events ourselves, both marathons and cancer treatments, we were inspired by Dean's accomplishments.

Virginia began to read, "It was approaching midnight as I wove up the deserted road..." As the pain diminished and my mind cleared, she asked me, "What are we in now?" I answered that we were in just another marathon. "Right," she said, "and just as we have gotten through all the others, we are going to get through this one."

The year and a half following my surgery was full of challenges. I received a course of radiation in my hip and then entered a clinical trial for an experimental drug, ipilimumab. It caused a massive case of sarcoidosis that left lumps inside and outside my body. I then had surgery to prove that the lumps between my lungs were not melanoma. During all this time, I trained for the Los Angeles Marathon with a wonderful coach, Katie Curran. I managed some half marathons as training, but the March 4, 2007 Los Angeles Marathon proved too much and my weakened body collapsed at mile eighteen. Surviving the effects of ipilimumab and doing the 2008 marathon then became obsessions.

Virginia decided that the 2008 Los Angeles Marathon should be mine alone and that she would be my support. On March 2, I lined up with 25,000 other people and then we all surged forward to the sound of "We Love LA," some to prove they were strong, some to show they were beautiful, and me to prove I had endured.

We planned that I would run and walk the first twenty-two miles and then meet Virginia, who would cover the last four miles with me. This was strategic because it was here where I would generally begin to crack physically and psychologically. One hundred feet from mile marker twenty-two I could see her, peanut butter sandwich in hand and beautiful smile on her face. Four miles to go and through it all I would have a beautiful woman at my side.

Virginia made sure I kept my concentration and my pace. "Step it up Van," she ordered. I stepped it up.

Coach Katie called Virginia and asked how I was doing. "OK," Virginia answered.

"Is he leaning?" she asked.

"No, he is strong and straight and even carrying on a conversation." Virginia answered.

"Are you sure it's Van?" Katie joked.

"Step up the pace, Van," Virginia again ordered. I stepped up the pace. At mile twenty-five, there was Coach Katie in person waiting with a smile.

"How you doing Van?" I heard.

I asked her, "Is that the finish line on that banner ahead? I can't read it."

"No," Katie responded. "That is the banner for mile twenty-six. After that you have to turn right and the finish is .2 miles away."

"It's not the finish?" I asked.

"No. It is not."

I passed mile twenty-six. We turned to the right. I blurted out, "I see the finish."

"Do you want to run in, Van?" Katie asked.

"I can't," I gasped. "I have big blisters on my feet. I'll bust them if I run."

"OK, are you sure?" both Virginia and Katie prodded.

I made a lunge and stopped.

"He wants to," I heard Virginia say, and then I ran. I ran for my life.

1.

My God. How Did This Happen?

Chronic Myelogenous Leukemia
August 1997

The events that led to Virginia's diagnosis of chronic myelogenous leukemia (CML) began in Africa. As a dean at Cal Poly Pomona in California, I was responsible for a number of economic development programs in Zimbabwe and we would travel there on occasion, sometimes adding a few days of personal vacation. The rigors of a fast-paced trip masked the fact that Virginia had health problems.

We had started in Johannesburg, where we met with Citibank officials about funding in Zimbabwe a program similar to one Citibank and Cal Poly had instituted in Vietnam. After the meeting, we beelined it to the airport where we picked up a car and drove 300 miles late into the night to get to Kruger National Park. I had driven in unlighted backcountry before, but people streaming along both sides of the road loaded with bags and with children in their arms, made the trip unusually stressful. The park and its animals were awe-inspiring from a distance. We were both taken aback, though, when a huge baboon jumped on the hood of the car in front of us, grabbed the windshield wipers, and refused to dismount. When a thorn punctured my tire and I had to get out to change the spare, I kept looking over my shoulder for something that might eat me. In fact, I was so freaked I left my glasses on the top of my car. We still picture a very stylish baboon wearing them.

Two days later, we drove back to Johannesburg to catch a plane to Harare, Zimbabwe, where we met with the local director of the Kellogg Foundation about a food security program we were proposing for the rural areas. We then met with government officials. After that, we caught a small plane to a remote game camp known as Chizarira. There we walked twice a day among the elephants, hyenas, zebras, gazelles, Cape buffalo, and various scary cats. After two days we were back in Harare for a conference and more meetings all over the city. Zimbabwe was a wonderful place to visit, and our friends and colleagues made sure we were busy seeing every part of it.

Through all of this, Virginia was getting uncharacteristically tired. An aerobics fanatic, she had been in good shape as long as I had known her. I began to wonder if something was wrong when her fatigue forced her to turn down an exotic trip to Nyanga in the highlands. Some sort of mass had developed just under her rib cage. She experienced night sweats that soaked our sheets. Her appetite disappeared and she lost weight. We tried to explain her fatigue as a product of the rigors of travel and meetings, her night sweats as menopause, the weight loss as a diet she had been on for the previous few months, and the lump as traveler's constipation. By the time we departed Zimbabwe, though, we knew Virginia had to discuss these problems with her doctor.

Virginia, who rarely saw a doctor for more than an annual physical, told her doctor about the symptoms. The doctor recommended a blood test and an ultrasound a few days after. Virginia dutifully took the doctor's referrals. The doctor could see that Virginia was in very big trouble, but she hadn't told her patient.

It was at this time that Virginia, who had been an avid journaler since 1972, began chronicling her experience and feelings.

August 6, 1997: I am sitting on the bed when the phone rings. I answer it.

Doctor: Your blood test came back abnormal.

Me: Oh really?

Doctor: Yes. You have chronic myelogenous leukemia.

Me: Chronic what?

Doctor: Chronic myelogenous leukemia.

Me: Oh.

Doctor: Do you want me to spell it?

Me: Yes.

Doctor: C-h-r-o-n-i-c—————

Me: Thanks.

Doctor: Are you OK?

Me: Sure.

Doctor: I need you to come in because I have a referral to the oncologist. But have your husband drive you.

Me: OK.

August 6, 1997: Today was the beginning of my awareness of the disease running rampant in me. So many thoughts and emotions swirled in my head, I couldn't even identify them. This day begins a chain of events that is beyond what I always knew as reality.

Virginia called me at work. "Van, the doctor says I have chronic myelogenous leukemia." I was a seasoned dean at Cal Poly Pomona, but that didn't stop me from walking into the office of my assistant Kim, who had spent her professional life saving my butt and guiding me toward success, and muttering, "Virginia has leukemia," and then breaking down.

What exactly was wrong with her? What a jerk that doctor was to tell her over the phone. Were we going to have to deal with jerks like that? Does her doctor know what she is talking about? What was going to happen to her? What was going to happen to me? Could she work? Could I work? What would happen to our finances? Could she beat this thing? If not, what would happen to me? Would I be lonely? What must she be feeling? Was there a way to fight? Maybe this was a mistake. How could we find out? Why did this have to happen to her? She was always so healthy. Why did this have to happen to her, to me? How would we tell people? How would we tell her mother? These thoughts swarmed inside my head, followed by the guilt that said they were selfish.

Although ignorant as to the beast we were facing, we would have to make major decisions quickly. I felt fear—the full-blown terror that comes when something rips your life from end to end. This was black, black terror. My new universe had been created.

Neither of us remembers much from the post-diagnosis meeting with the doctor. Virginia remembers asking her to again spell chronic myelogenous leukemia. She remembers the doctor saying "think cure" and talking about a bone marrow transplant. I remember she told us that this was a terminal disease and that Virginia might live three to five years. In trying to spell the disease, we were grasping to absorb its meaning, its power.

Virginia's white cell count was very high, as were her platelet and basophil counts. We knew things looked bad, but despite the diagnosis, we had yet to be convinced that Virginia had CML. I called my friends in Zimbabwe to see if their doctors had ever seen blood counts like Virginia's associated with any sort of local diseases. I was hoping for malaria. Can you imagine? No, they told me. It was very likely that Virginia had leukemia.

Even in her weakened state, Virginia fought for her rights as a patient and sought out specialists. Luckily, my assistant Kim came through with her sister-in-law's referral to one of the best oncologists in our area, Dr. Douglas Blayney. We see Kim's sister-in-law, Gail, from time to time and we always thank her for her help in guiding us to someone who knew what he was doing. With him, we thought we had a chance to save Virginia's life.

Although the doctors had been delivering the bad news with certainty, in order to be sure Virginia had leukemia, she had to subject herself to a bone marrow aspiration and biopsy. In this procedure, a hollow corkscrew-like device is used to drill a hole in the upper part of the hip where the pelvic bone is closest to the surface. Once the hole is drilled through the bone and into the marrow, samples of the marrow and bone are extracted up the center of the corkscrew and then sent off for analysis. Though Dr. Blayney tried to lighten the mood by telling us that it would be OK because he had just watched the training video, the process was unthinkably painful.

Virginia would ultimately have fourteen such procedures. She never cried out; from that moment, she was already displaying the strength she would need to survive.

August 8, 1997: I'm walking into a CANCER center on August 8 with Van. I can't believe I'm doing this. I'm carrying a copy of my blood work. Dr. Blayney, Gail, Nancy (nurse), Myra (nurse), and Rose and Terry (receptionists) introduce themselves. They are so sweet and kind it makes me cry.

Dr. Blayney, who seems very personable, says he thinks I have acute myelogenous leukemia and that I'll be in the hospital with a shunt in my chest for chemotherapy—I won't be returning to work. My heart pounds as it begins to register that I'm nearly a goner.

I can't get words out without bursting into tears. I'm having a bone marrow extraction and biopsy. I'm on my stomach, and I'm hurting. Van stays to hold my hand. Gail holds my other hand. I am deeply touched amid my pain.

It took a while to get the results from the lab—longer than it should have and longer than we had time for. As we waited, Virginia's white count began to shoot up. As it did, the lump, which turned out to be her swollen spleen, grew correspondingly. When the count reached fifteen times the high normal count of 10.8 and was rising by twenty points a day and her platelets were twice the high normal of 400, Dr. Blayney decided to treat her with the traditional treatment for CML, hydroxyurea. If Virginia did indeed have CML, her white count would fall in response. He explained that hydroxyurea would bring Virginia's health back to an approximation of normal. Her white counts would drop and her spleen would shrink, but it would have no effect on the progression of the disease. At minimum, it gave us time to get confirming blood tests and decide what we should try as an alternative.

August 12, 1997: The weekend comes, and the pain of not knowing exactly what I have continues. After two days of spiritual agony, I return to Dr. Blayney's office to be told I have chronic myelogenous leukemia, not acute. I can go back to work! I never thought I'd be thankful to return to my job after the summer is over, but now I cherish the opportunity.

Worldwide, close to 10,000 people annually are newly diagnosed with chronic myelogenous leukemia—4,500 of them in the United States. At the time of Virginia's diagnosis, 35,000 people with CML were alive worldwide, and close to 18,000 of them were in the United

States. As Dr. Blayney explained, CML was a very rare type of cancer—almost always fatal, with the life expectancy typically three to five years after diagnosis. The only proven cure was a bone marrow transplant. But this was an unlikely option for Virginia since she had no siblings to match her marrow and she was fifty-one years old, older than most transplant centers would help at that time.

Then Dr. Blayney told us that there was another relatively new drug called interferon that might fend off the CML. It was designed to stimulate the body's immune system and thus help it to recognize and kill the cancer cells. Dr. Blayney recommended we try it while we pursued a donor for a bone marrow transplant. He explained that without the bone marrow transplant or interferon, Virginia's only alternative would be to take the hydroxyurea, and within a few years she would enter advanced stage CML. At this phase, her white cell count would begin to soar. These young cells would reproduce and take over the marrow. Called blasts, they would be too young to effectively fight off any type of infection. In the early advanced stage, Virginia might have six months to a year before she entered the phase of the disease called blast crisis, where her chromosomes would be under attack. As her genome was hacked to pieces, her body's ability to repair the damage would be gone. She might also have very high platelet counts but a dysfunctional clotting system. In blast crisis, she would die in short order either from some opportunistic infection or spontaneous bleeding. We read gruesome descriptions of people dying with blood seeping out of every orifice. The fact was that we had no idea how long Virginia had had CML because her doctor had never taken blood tests during past physicals. She might have been on the edge of blast crisis when she was first diagnosed. We will never know. This realization reinforced the conclusion that our only bet was on interferon. We accepted Dr. Blayney's advice. Virginia started interferon.

Dr. Blayney told us that interferon would make Virginia feel like she had a mild case of the flu. It would soon become obvious that the experience would be a lot worse than a bout with the flu.

August 12, 1997: What is to become of me? Will I die soon? Why did I get this disease? I look after my health, I work out, I eat right; I've been so healthy. Where is the justice? These thoughts bump around in my head for a while until I admit they are counterproductive.

Borders Bookstore: $140 on books about cancer and cancer survivors.

Home: I begin to read avidly. Van begins to learn the ins and outs of the Internet. We fill three four-inch binders with information from chat room talk to journal articles to drug info. I find I can't read them because they upset my outlook. So Van becomes my "research guy" and turns into a compulsive computer guy, staying up till 3 a.m. and dragging himself to work.

I wondered who we should tell about Virginia's disease. Virginia, who is by nature open, took care of any decision by telling just about anyone who wanted to listen that she had leukemia. I came to realize the wisdom of this approach. When people learned that Virginia had leukemia, they often were able to offer help.

An early example of this help following openness came when I told my neighbor Bud McAndrew about Virginia's diagnosis. Bud is a down-to-earth fellow who knows a lot about computers. He asked me if I knew very much about the disease. I must have shown my profound ignorance—and genuine fear—in response. He sat me down and showed me how to do research on the Web.

I have a Ph.D. in history, but it had been a while since I had done serious research. Furthermore, I was of the pre-Google generation. I can never thank my friend Bud enough for opening up a world that ultimately helped us find the one solution that saved Virginia's life.

I was never better at anything than the CML research. I often thought that this was what my career in higher education had prepared me for. Not only could I research, but my position as dean afforded me access to many knowledgeable academics and experts who could fill in the technical gaps. The knowledge I gained and my ability to learn came to define my relationship with the medical community. I came to realize that those in the medical profession will do their best to inform you to a basic level, but unless you show an interest and capacity to understand, they won't go beyond that. And simplistic summaries are not really useful in a search for lifesaving answers. So, I began to read.

The history of chronic myelogenous leukemia is fascinating. In 1960, Philadelphia scientists Peter Nowell and David Hungerford discovered that cells from patients with CML had a shortened chromosome 22. It was the first time it appeared clear that a specific disease was associated with a chromosomal abnormality. This aberrant chromosome soon came to be known as the Philadelphia chromosome in reference to the place of its discovery. By 1960, no one was yet able to identify individual genes, and so there remained a mystery about where the piece of chromosome 22 actually went; but the identity of the Philadelphia chromosome opened the door to more research into the connection between this chromosomal abnormality and CML.

With further improvements in chromosomal imaging, and the ability to identify specific genes, scientists in the 1970s discovered that chromosome 22 broke at a gene called BCR while chromosome 9 broke in the middle of a gene known as ABL, and they exchanged material. The reciprocal translocation created a new part to chromosome 22 called the BCR-ABL fusion gene, or the Philadelphia + chromosome. It was shorter because it came out with less material in the exchange. This was the source of CML, but how was this associated with the origin and pathology of CML? In the '80s David Baltimore of MIT, his post doc, Owen Witte, and others found that the real culprit was the incomplete part of ABL that was attached to chromosome 22. A healthy ABL's function was to switch on and order the production of new white cells when needed, and then to turn off when that was accomplished. The problem was that when ABL broke free on chromosome 9, it left behind all its control circuitry. Missing its controls, the part of ABL that attached to chromosome 22 ordered the full-tilt production of white cells and never turned off. In other words, the cells with the BCR-ABL abnormality would reproduce constantly. Moreover, these aberrant cells received no instructions to die as normal cells would. Owen Witte moved to UCLA but continued to work with Baltimore and his other colleagues to work out the precise way the BCR-ABL gene did its damage.

BCR-ABL, like normal genes, is basically a formula that is read by a complicated process and then translated into a corresponding protein that does its assigned business in the body. ABL as it normally functions creates a protein known as a tyrosine kinase, whose function is to take on energy and then use it to send a message from one part of the cell to another. Under certain environmental conditions the protein will change shape slightly, opening up a pocket that invites an Adenosine 5'-triphosphate (ATP) molecule to attach. Then it captures a phosphate from ATP that charges the protein in a process called phosphorylation. With a charge, the ABL protein can send a message (called signal transduction) to the cell that then multiplies. When the job is done, the protein resumes its original shape, leaving no pocket to accept ATP. In the BCR-ABL cells, the pocket is always receptive to ATP and rampant Philadelphia positive (PH+) white cell production begins overwhelming the normal cells. With reproduction high, the white cells become progressively younger and less able to do what mature leukocytes do. Within a few years these young cells (blasts) become more common and crowded in the blood stream until they are basically all that are left and the patient enters into blast crisis and dies. In 1990, scientists induced CML in mice by injecting BCR-ABL into them in a study that proved definitively that BCR-ABL was the source of CML. This was the multi-lettered monster we were facing.

David Baltimore later became president of Cal Tech and at a business meeting I was able to thank him for the part he had he played in moving CML research forward. For his part, he was glad to see the face of a person he had helped.

With my educational background, I mastered Internet research rather quickly. Still, the process itself was tedious and time-consuming. As I sought out the best medical care, a large teaching and research hospital seemed the answer. For us in Los Angeles, that meant UCLA or USC.

The answer came to me in a grocery aisle—a place I hadn't frequented for several decades, but had to now, as it was all Virginia could do to get to work and home again. Wheeling down one of the aisles, my mind focused on my research, I literally ran into someone's stomach with my cart. I looked up and found I had rammed Tani Welch, a long-time friend. For several of the ten years we had known her, her husband Colin was being treated at Jonsson Cancer Center at UCLA for a large tumor behind his left eye. Amazingly, he had survived seven years with surgery after surgery and brilliant care, though the price they had paid was constant travel to UCLA. Not caring about the shoppers wheeling by in this very public place, I broke down as I told my friend what had happened to Virginia. Tani later told me that all I had in my shopping cart was beer, a lot of beer. I asked her, "You mean like a six pack?" She laughed, "No, a lot more than that!" She told me Colin was doing pretty well and that they were going to UCLA the next day. Then it dawned on me to ask her to ask his doctor who was the best leukemia person at UCLA. The next day Colin asked his doctor, "If your wife had leukemia, who would you go to?" Colin has since passed on, but I can still thank him for such a clever way to ask my question. The answer was Dr. Mary Territo, who was head of the bone marrow transplant unit at UCLA's Jonsson Cancer Center. We heard from Tani and Colin that night, and we made an appointment the next day. We were now entering the world of a teaching and research hospital, bringing with us renewed hope. We had entered not only the world of Dr. Mary Territo, but also that of Dr. Owen Witte, who was then at UCLA, and all the other bright researchers who sought work at UCLA to learn from him and who would eventually present an answer for Virginia.

I vividly remember the waiting room as we waited to see Dr. Territo. To me it seemed jammed with suffering people without hair, people with disfigurements and very thin, very, very quiet cancer patients. Over the years, I would learn a lot about the heroics of the people I saw, but on that day they scared the hell out of me. I wanted to run. Would Virginia be like that? The answer was yes, and she would be as heroic as them too.

Dr. Territo, being head of the transplant unit, began to talk to us about this possibility for Virginia. She signed Virginia up for the bone marrow transplant registry and initiated a search for an unrelated donor.

She had us read the provided summary of processes and risks associated with bone marrow transplants. Another shock. Like most people, we assumed those who contracted cancer got a bone marrow transplant, waited for it to work, and then went on to live long and productive lives. What we found was that even if Virginia were to have a transplant, the odds would not be very good. At best, there was a 50 percent chance she would be dead in the first thirty days. Lucky for us, Dr. Territo did not push and almost incidentally mentioned that there was CML research going on at UCLA that looked very promising. Little did we know at the time that this little piece of information would be part of Virginia's survival.

August 14, 1997: UCLA Medical Center: I register, fill out forms, deal with the short, curt manner of the clerk, and wait amid maimed and white, pasty-faced other patients. Finally we are escorted to Dr. Territo's examination room. Van's sister Connie and my best friend Judy Dunbridge stay in the waiting room.

Dr. Territo: May I have your papers and slides? I need to look at them now.

Me: Here they are.

We wait in that room for forty-five more minutes when Mary Territo returns and concurs I have CML.

Dr. Territo: What do you know about this disease?

Me: It's caused by a Philadelphia chromosome that breaks off. Most people last two to three years then convert to acute stage and die. Bone marrow transplant is not optimal treatment for me as I have no siblings.

Dr. Territo: Well, you know quite a bit! Hopefully you'll never have to have a BMT because of a new drug being studied in a lab here at UCLA that's showing great promise for success in treating CML. The researchers hope to get FDA approval to study it in humans in a year.

I left UCLA feeling the first real hope since August 6.

Back at home, I delved directly into research on bone marrow transplants. I first found out that if you are going to have a transplant, you want to be young. In those days very few people were transplanted at Virginia's age, older than 50, because it was felt that they were probably not strong enough to stand up to the rigors of what was involved. Furthermore, you wanted to have a perfect match. Barring that, there was a strong chance that the new marrow would wreak havoc in the patient's body, and the new marrow might out-survive the patient. I was willing to go along with whatever Virginia wanted, but also terrified that she would say, let's chance it. Luckily, she shared my misgivings, though she wanted to stay on the registry until fate forced her to make a decision. That time came in June 1998 when Dr. Territo told her that she had found a preliminary match. Did she want to go forward? Exhaling a deep breath, she said no. The moment reinforced the fact that our decisions from that day on would be life-and-death ones. Before this experience, we assumed most medical procedures go from point A to a fix. We learned that in cancer treatments, you often go from point A to death, and certainly that was the case for transplants. In our ripe young fifties, we had gone from making decisions about where to eat to whether to risk death in thirty days.

Dr. Blayney now needed to know if a transplant was going to be Virginia's choice. The answer was definitely no. We were now totally committed to interferon.

I read everything I could find about interferon. The most fascinating was the book *A Commotion in the Blood,* which chronicled the discovery and development of the drug.

As it turned out, Dr. Blayney was right to recommend interferon. It causes too much damage to be a long-term solution to any disease, but I am convinced today that it bought Virginia survival time and me time to research other options. It was time for Virginia to really suffer.

2.

Interferon and ARA-C

A Year from Hell

A month after diagnosis, Virginia began her interferon treatment by going to the doctor's office every day to get an injection of eight million units of interferon alpha. The standard treatments for hepatitis C and melanoma are 3 million units three days a week, so this was by comparison a very big dose. After her first shot she went home, directly to the toilet and threw up. Next she fell asleep, sweated all night, woke up in the morning with a fever, and was as ill as she could ever remember. Then she sucked it up and went to work. After work she went back to the cancer center and got another 8 mu shot, tried to eat something, graded school papers, and went to bed. Other than trading the vomiting for constant nausea and ultimately learning to inject herself, this would be Virginia's routine for a year.

One morning she awoke to a fistful of hair on her pillow. Soon she looked like a semi-balding little old lady. She tried on wigs, even bought and styled one, but they hurt and she gave up on them. Her weight dropped quickly from 140 to 102 pounds. I tried to find tricks to make her eat. "Here is the airplane. Open up the hangar" was not well received. I finally found tapioca pudding, but a person cannot live on tapioca pudding. She was such a sad-looking little thing. Actually it was frightening. Then I made things worse.

Through my desperate studies, I had learned that research in France showed that the addition of a drug called cytarabine or ARA-C to interferon was more effective in treating CML than interferon alone. We talked to Dr. Blayney about adding ARA-C to the interferon. Another bone marrow aspiration and biopsy made it clear that we were not getting results from the interferon alone, so he said, "Why not?"

This added another drug to the mix and another injection to Virginia's nightly interferon regimen. For all the effort we saw no improvement; and worse, mouth sores began to erupt. The pain was so great that Virginia couldn't eat solid food. I learned you can liquefy just about anything. But even the pureed food was painful to swallow. She ate as much as she possibly could. It got so bad that she couldn't talk. Being a high school English teacher, Virginia found this devastating; effectively, it meant she couldn't teach. Eventually, yet another medicine made it possible for her to talk and teach, but she had to rest in the parking lot before she could make it all the way to her classroom. Through all this, Virginia was willing to do whatever it took to stay alive. But despite her strong will, things were to get worse. Soon, she would be challenged to the limit.

October 15, 1997: After four and a half weeks on the chemotherapy, I am still kickin'. It is very hard to get up and going in the morning, and I feel "shaky," kind of like a hangover. Most days I just don't feel quite right. At night, I fall fast asleep by 8 p.m. This is quite frustrating as I used to be a semi-night owl.

Sunday night I went to dinner with Van and an associate dean candidate and his wife plus Eric and Gloria McLaughlin. I could barely stay awake—it is so difficult. I know I have to do what I have to do, but I am getting impatient with all this sleeping.

I'm on my second round of ARA-C (ten days on, eighteen days off) and so far, so good.

October 15—4:15 p.m.

Dr. Blayney: How are things?

Me: Great!

Dr. Blayney: Really?

Me: Really!

Dr. Blayney? Are you working? Miss any days?

Me: Yes, yes, one day because I couldn't talk because of my mouth sore.

Dr. Blayney: You look pretty good.

Me: I'm just tired a lot of the time, especially in the a.m. when I get up.

Dr. Blayney: That should either pass or diminish with time.

Me: (Thank God he said that.)

October 24, 1997: School is going fairly well. It is very hard to get up and get going in the mornings. I feel shaky and sooo so tired. Walking into the building is extremely taxing and my steps are very slow. But I do it. I put one foot in front of the other and before I know it, I am in my room.

Kids are so sweet. One day last week, a sophomore came up to my table on her way out and said, "Mrs. Garner, I know it's hard for you right now, but I want you to know that I admire you and that I know everything will be all right." I was so touched I had to struggle to keep back tears. This is why it is worth it for me to come every day I can. I have only missed one day, when I had a mouth sore that was so bad I couldn't talk. I got to school but had to get Susan to call for a sub. I guess this is pretty good considering my situation.

Each day I leave school at about 3:00 p.m. and get home, give myself two shots and take a nap. If I have to go to the cancer care center, I don't get home until four or four thirty, but I do a lot of sleeping. By 8:00 p.m., I am asleep for the night. I am getting tired of this routine—I get next to nothing accomplished. The house is a veritable mess, although Van is contributing to keeping it neater. He gets up with me each morning and fixes me something to eat as well as a cup of coffee to take with me. He also fixes me something to eat at night and cleans up the kitchen before he goes to bed. He has become my savior. He makes sure I do eat, because most of the time I don't care if I do or not. I went to Nordstrom to buy some pants because all of mine are so large, and I had to get a size 2 in one pair. I guess I must look thinner than I think I do.

I haven't been going to aerobics on a regular basis—too tired, and I'm on too much of a weird schedule with the injections I get every day. When I go to the cancer center to get them, the time is not right for aerobics. I worry about my muscles; all that work I have done to tone myself up—I don't want it to go to waste. I do go when I can, and then I am only on the step—no risers at all. Even then it is hard. But my friends have been so sweet. Kenny, a very large African-American guy who used to walk with us and who is a custodian at Ganesha High School, threw his arms around me Wednesday night and kissed me on the cheek. He was worried about me because I had not been to work out for a week. Marietta, a fellow walker and sweet lady who bicycles in long rides, calls me to see how I am and sets up a step for me in case I am late. Everyone is very concerned and I am touched by this, too.

I'm not sure, but I think my hair is thinning out. I didn't expect this to happen so fast. I thought it happened only to people who have been on the drug for a long time. I guess time will tell. I hope that all this is working toward my disease being controlled and that I am headed toward cytogenetic remission, meaning the Philadelphia chromosome disappears from my blood and bone marrow. It will be a while before we can find this out. I have just completed a second round of ARA-C and have another mouth sore just like the first round. Same place, just not as bad. I am on interferon and ARA-C for ten days and then just interferon for eighteen days. It is turning out to be not so bad, but there are all these things that change my life. I am supposed to be used to the drugs and not feel so tired eventually. I wish it would happen soon.

In all of this, Virginia's friends and family cried silently for her, but never showed it. My sister and our nephews, Stephen and Craig, met us for breakfast Sunday after Sunday. One day Virginia heard the youngest boy, Craig, ask his mother if leukemia was catching. That little boy was willing to go to breakfast with Virginia, week after week, seeing her pathetic state, without knowing if he might catch her disease. We love those boys. Virginia was beginning to get visits by an increasing number of friends. We finally figured out that they thought she was dying and wanted to see her before she passed away.

As hard as we were fighting, I knew they were right. Virginia was dying.

Her mind was also getting foggier. Her best friend found ways not to ride in a car with her. She certainly scared me. We call it the "oops" period of driving because one day parking at UCLA, she misjudged her parking skills and crunched the hubcap of the car next to her. I looked over at her; she looked over at me, smiled, and said "oops" in the most endearing way. This was neither the last nor the worst incident with an automobile.

November 10, 1997: I have begun to shed my hair like crazy. I can reach up and grab a handful of hair, pull, and several strands come out. When I wash it, there are gobs in the sink. This is something I hadn't planned on. What will I eventually look like? Will it be really noticeable? I know I can't wear a wig for the rest of my life. I don't think I could for even a few weeks. I also have developed really dry skin—everywhere. Nothing helps. Although sometimes not as bad, fatigue assails me. I have no appetite, and I have shrunk to 115 pounds. I force myself to eat and drink either Boost or Ensure Plus.

Although we still keep a social calendar, I find myself impatient with the socializing. Really all I want to do is lie down and read or watch TV—a sad commentary and sharp contrast to my former self. It is alarming to me at times to think about, but I've decided I have to accept and to realize this may not be a permanent thing.

Van continues to be my savior. Without him I'm not sure I'd be eating at all. He does most grocery shopping and cooking. He keeps track of me and my food intake. He fixes something for me to eat each morning at 6 a.m. He loves me no matter what. How lucky can I be?

I dug into my research more desperately every day. It seemed obvious Virginia needed something else. Periodic bone marrow tests were still showing 100 percent leukemia cells. Researchers were experimenting with just about every drug and combination of drugs possible. The problem was not so much finding something to try; it was finding the thing with the best prospects. With Virginia as sick as she was becoming, we knew she had one shot left.

November 25, 1997: The past couple of weeks have been rough. My hair is coming out faster and faster, and my scalp is visible through it now. Every time I wash my hair, I dread looking in the drain. Every time

I comb and blow-dry my hair, I cringe at the loose hairs that come out. Who knows how much more will be lost? The doctor and nurses say it's the ARA-C that's causing it. I guess that means that all my hair could fall out since I'm on ARA-C forever. The rest of my hair has stopped growing. When I went to the hairdresser, she didn't even cut it. I also think my eyelashes and eyebrows have lost hair.

Since I'm a "hair person," this has been emotionally extremely difficult for me. I will get a wig, but I want it to be a really good and comfortable one. Having to wear a wig for the rest of my life is not my idea of having a good time—but then neither is having no appetite/ forcing myself to eat or sleeping from 6 p.m. to 5:30 a.m. because of the severe fatigue—or getting canker sores ten days a month. If I let myself, I could get really depressed. My existence is day-to-day and sometimes that is very hard.

I am still at work and things are going OK, but I know I don't have the usual perkiness I used to have. I try my best.

Sometimes I feel like I'm very tired and want to rest. I can't even concentrate to read. Actually I feel "itchy"—unable to sit still—but I can feel better if I lie down. It's very odd and hard to get used to. I wish I could be the way I used to be. I wish I could feel good for a while. Maybe this will happen to me eventually. I can only say it will and move forward. What a gift it would be. To have some joy in eating would also be nice. Forcing myself to eat is getting harder and harder. What joy to "wolf down" food and have it taste good (or even just not to be on the verge of gagging)!

The most frustrating thing about searching out clinical trials is that many, many honest hardworking people are out there making cogent arguments maintaining their approach makes sense and the others do not. In fact, in cancer research, it is very likely that no one is totally right. To find out, you have to look at everything from a scientific as well as a historical perspective. A concept makes sense. So you ask, has anyone ever made it work? If nothing has yet worked, then what makes the most sense? What did the animal studies reveal? Is a big company behind it?

December 1, 1997: Beginnings—

All day I felt extremely wired—like I had had twenty cups of coffee. I couldn't sit still while waiting for my food to arrive at a restaurant.

My heart races when I walk or exert myself.

I don't want to socialize—it just seems like too much effort.

December 8, 1997: I am doing much better now. I am able to eat and enjoy it. I've kept up with the little things in life like paying bills, and we put up the lights outside and got our Xmas tree in the house yesterday. I've ordered a wig and it should be done by Friday. Shellie will style it so it looks like my own hair. We'll see. School is going fine—I'm keeping up but sometimes I wonder how!

I find little patience with socializing with people. I don't even like talking on the phone. I don't know why. Also, I can't stand the wait for food in a restaurant—worse than normal. These are phenomena I can't explain and that are new to me.

At school today, the women held a "hat day" in solidarity with my thinning hair. It was so sweet when they told me last week, I cried.

Life moves on…and today I launched back into ARA-C. Oh well.

Every day I have to try so hard just to get through. Eating, fatigue, ignoring my temptation to wish I could be well—it's very wearing on a person. Even on a good day, I have to try so hard.

December 18, 1997: New development: thrush in my mouth. Worst canker sore ever—stayed home from school Monday. The pain was incessant and excruciating. I've been eating by drinking blender drinks of baby food meat and green beans. The doctor gave me these prescriptions:

Iron three times a day.

Medicine for the thrush.

Acyclovir for the canker sore.

So I am really a pill junkie now!

My hemoglobin is way up, so at least I feel better! I got some Christmas shopping done yesterday, and I feel good about that!

From the beginning, Virginia experienced the love and kindness of her students. On January 2, 1998 Charles Ro wrote and then gave Virginia the following parody of *Hamlet*:

Keep on, Virginia
Your name is hardly frailty
Strength is what sets you apart.
Even in the midst of hell and chemicals
You find the strength to share
You find the strength to live
And your body ails, your mind is weary
But you allow yourself no other choice
But to continue for those who need you.
For all of those who pass you off as weak
For a society that has deemed you a "citizen"
You bear the burden of 1,000 heroes, 41 presidents,
And yet smile at the end of a rough day.
There are no accolades or jackpots in the form of checks
And too often are you cursed and overlooked
But if we had more sense to realize your value
We should crown you as our queen of strength,
Of beauty, and only smile at the thought of
Your example.
Keep on Virginia, keep on.
Charles Ro
1/2/98

As Virginia kept on, I kept on researching, and I was beginning to question the biases of the particular pharmaceutical companies. Some of these are driven by what I call a salvage mentality. How do you drop a drug after you have put 25 million dollars into its development and testing? The answer I kept finding? To preserve investments, you don't. Researchers dedicate their entire careers to developing approaches to particular diseases and to drugs that support those approaches. Some doctors recommend clinical trials that have very little prospect for success, perhaps to fill a trial of theirs or of their colleagues because it is remunerative and enhances professional credentials. Filling a trial is a prerequisite to running one. As a person who has benefited tremendously from two clinical trials, I still give this warning.

I also advise people to look at results. All clinical trials have results published somewhere. You will find results where investigators say that they find that an investigational drug shows no benefit to the targeted group. You may find that very small numbers benefited. You may find that the benefit is not that much and you may also find that the benefits are not worth what it does to the quality of life. Some drugs are quite nasty. Still, you or your loved one may have his or her back to the wall. All other treatments have failed, and the will to live forces you forward. You do your damnedest to ferret out the best trial.

January 13, 1998: Over Winter Break, I began to feel much better. By the first week back at work I was eating well and feeling well. I went to aerobics twice last week! I'm back on ARA-C (the second week) and have my sores in my mouth but they're not as bad as last time. Perhaps the acyclovir is helping ameliorate the problem.

Yesterday I went to UCLA and had a bone marrow biopsy. My appointment was at 1 p.m. I got out of there at 4:30 p.m. It was all waiting—I was questioned on things I'd answered before by a young doctor who is a fellow for Dr. Territo. Saw Dr. Territo for three minutes. The "fellow" gave me a bone marrow biopsy. It wasn't too bad, but it hurt like last time. Today I'm pretty sore. But I feel pretty good, actually. Three more days of ARA-C, then I can feel even better.

Virginia couldn't see the young doctor's face when he was doing the bone marrow biopsy. This was obviously something he had never done before and he was sweating profusely. He hurt Virginia a lot more than she remembers and she bled a lot. When we discussed with a nurse what had happened, she told us that we had the right to refuse treatment by anyone and demand that Dr. Territo do the bone marrow biopsies. Although they tried, we never again let a resident or fellow practice on Virginia.

I want to feel normal. I'd give anything to be in that spot. I want to gain five to seven pounds so I can wear most of my clothes, and I want my hair to grow back. But most of all, I want to live a long and happy life. I hope the bone marrow biopsy (BMB) shows some response to the protocol. It would give me a great boost.

Sometimes I get down about how my life has changed and how it will be that way indefinitely. But I try to deal with reality by looking for positives, and generally that helps. One of the biggest—actually the biggest—positives is my dear, dear husband, Van. Yesterday when I thought insanity would descend while going through all that waiting, he bolstered me up. During the procedure, he held my hand and allowed me to squeeze his. I'm sure I drained his fingers of circulation. He is a sweet and very special man. I'm so fortunate he loves me.

January 14, 1998: Today is a hard day. My mouth sore is so bad I have trouble talking, eating, and drinking. I'm really becoming weary of dealing with this, but I guess I'm stuck for quite a while. My back hurts where they did the bone marrow biopsy—I keep forgetting and leaning up against things.

I think if there were something that would help my mouth, my life would be so much better. Too bad there isn't. It is very depressing to know that just as I start to feel good again, it's time to go back on the ARA-C and get mouth sores. But I must continue to give myself the best possible chance to be saved.

So far I haven't had to take much work home. I seem to get it done at school. It makes me wonder what I'm doing differently this year. I don't think I've modified things too much. Students do work quietly at their tables while I grade papers, but they always did that. I relegate this to a mysterious phenomenon, but I'm glad of it.

Teaching seems to be getting a bit repetitive. Thinking about starting another spring semester creates an "oh not again." I guess this has nothing to do with my disease—probably a function of doing the same thing over and over for thirty years. Still, I'm happy to be able to do it because it means I am still alive and able to.

February 3, 1998: Yesterday I went for my monthly appointment with Dr. Blayney. Results from the bone marrow tests are still not back. Maybe they once again couldn't get a culture to grow. DB doesn't seem upset. I'm going to have a blood test today that tells the same thing.

He asked me if I'm depressed and I said I didn't really know. I did say I feel trapped in this protocol and that that in itself is depressing. He very compassionately told me it won't be forever. I'm not so sure. I guess we'll see.

My ear is still plugged up. I'm on my third round of antibiotics, but Van read that a side effect of interferon can be deafness. DB wants me to go to an ear nose and throat man just to make sure.

As of this week, my insurance company put a halt to taking filled syringes home from Wilshire Oncology. They say they don't want doctors to be drug dispensers. So Nancy ordered the drugs from a mail-order place and taught us how to draw up the interferon and to mix the ARA-C. This should bring quite a bit of freedom, although it makes me nervous. I know I'll get used to it.

There's always something!

February 6, 1998: Well loading my own syringes is nerve-racking, but I've managed to do it this week. I guess I'll gain more confidence as time goes on. It does give me much more freedom. My canker sores are back. They aren't too bad yet—I can still chew if I do it carefully. I wish it wouldn't get any worse. It's such a drag.

Van goes to Vietnam Sunday night for ten days. Mother is staying with me because I don't think I can do it myself. I need a cook and a cleaner. And a dog feeder. I am very concerned about how I'll do without Van. He is my absolute rock. I hope all goes smoothly.

February 10, 1998: Today is the ninth day of my ARA-C injections, and my canker sores are at their worst. I have discovered that it depends a lot on where (what physical location on my tongue) they are as to how bad they feel. This time they're way under toward the front, which seems to be less painful. I'm glad tomorrow is my last day!

Van called from Saigon last night. He made it safely and was off to a business lunch—no time to rest from the flight. Poor guy.

February 13, 1998: Sometimes I find myself wishing this would all go away and let me go back to my normal life. It's a wistful feeling and a luxury I can't allow myself to dwell on for too long. But the feelings are there and they cannot be denied. Maybe someday I'll be able to feel semi-normal at least. Living one day at a time can be hard, but it's the only way to keep a positive attitude.

February 18, 1998: Van comes home today. I am very glad because it's been very hard. My mother was a saint, but I know it practically did her in. She is glad to go home. Annie, our obstreperous little rescue dog, a small terrier mix, just about drove her nuts. Actually, she just about drives me nuts too. I talked to the vet about her whining to get out three times a night, and the vet said she should be able to hold it. I don't know, maybe she should sleep in the cage with the door shut. I don't know how long I can continue with this. But I get very sad when I think of finding another home for her. It's truly a difficult dilemma.

February 23, 1998: On Saturday, Van and I flew to San Jose. It was pouring rain—I've never seen rain like it; it was as if someone filled big buckets and dumped them on us, then went back to fill up the buckets again. We made it to our motel in Pacific Grove (next to Pebble Beach) in two hours. The wedding of John White, Van's old roommate, was at a church in Pebble Beach at 4 p.m. The reception was at a hotel in Pebble Beach at six and the dinner dance was from seven to midnight. I lasted until 11 p.m. and I even danced. It was fun to see our old friends. I know they all wonder about me and sometimes that makes me uncomfortable—but probably I'm being paranoid.

The truth was that by this time Virginia was down to 102 pounds and looked like a concentration camp survivor. Luckily she could not see herself that way and no one, including me, told her how sorrowful she looked.

Sunday morning we had breakfast with the our friends, (minus the bride and groom) in the hotel restaurant with an ocean view. The waves were absolutely gigantic. Good old El Nino. I did all right the whole time and I had worried I might not. So I feel good about that.

February 27, 1998: We finally got the results of my bone narrow biopsy, and it showed 100 percent Philadelphia chromosome. I knew this would depress me, but I also had known it was unlikely to be any different. The results showed no blasts though, which is good. Maybe by my test on April 6 there will be some change. I'm struggling to keep a positive outlook. I know I'm going to have to do something soon because I think I might be depressed. I'll talk to the doctor on Monday and see what he says. I seem to be missing some of the joy of life, and despair is hiding around the corner. I want to hold it back; I don't want to give in to it.

March 6, 1998: A lot has happened this week. I talked to Dr. Blayney about whether I am depressed or not and he gave these pills called Paxil, an antidepressant. After two pills, I was overcome with side effects—severe nausea, weak muscles, general dizziness, etc. I went home before sixth period on Wednesday and stayed home yesterday, sleeping the entire day. Van reads the paper that comes with the pills and found out these symptoms are common in 28 percent of the people who take these pills. Today I still don't feel normal—but then, what is normal anyway? At least I'm not nauseated anymore. Also I am taking the ARA-C and I do not have canker sores yet. Is it possible I may escape this time? What a wonderful occasion if so.

I had to find a solution to these mouth sores that I had inflicted on Virginia. My research finally paid off when I found that the problem was not unique and that the doctors at M.D. Anderson Cancer Center in Texas had just discovered the solution of lowering the overall dose of ARA-C and spreading out the injections from ten a month to every day. This change in the way we administered the ARA-C resulted in one of the few victories we would experience during those months, but it was a big one. Quality of life means a lot in the midst of a battle like this.

March 9, 1998: Still no canker sores! What a miracle, and how I appreciate it. It's heaven not worrying about my mouth. Van and I had a very nice weekend. We spent a lot of time together, and we had dinner on Saturday night with the Eaves and the McLaughlins. It was a relaxing weekend. Tonight Van and I are going to the CML support group to see what it's like.

The doctor gave me different pills for depression, but their side effects are even worse. I'll not take any pills for this right now.

March 10, 1998: Last night Van and I went to a support group I thought was strictly for CML patients but that we discovered was actually a blood cancer group. There were people there with multiple myeloma and non-Hodgkins lymphoma also. It was mostly an informational session—no whining, etc. I don't know if I'll go back because there wasn't much there for me. Vicki (the nurse) was there and the psychologist was named Gloria. She was very nice. I stayed up until 10 p.m. last night—a first for me in a long time! Maybe things are getting better.

Two more days of ARA-C. Still no mouth sores.

March 26, 1998: Much has happened since my last entry. I went to see the cancer center psychologist. She gave me the perspective that I may not be depressed—just mourning the old life I had. That made sense to me. I am sad when I think of what I've lost, and I'm scared when I think of the future—too many negative potentials. I do feel though that I will be healed. I am strong, and I have the best medical care, and I have a positive attitude. All these things in combination are good things going for me. I also have people praying for me all over the country. The power of prayer is proven.

On March 12, I stayed home because I had flu-like symptoms and had had a fever of 103.4 the night before. I wound up being home until March 24 because I had pneumonia. The oral antibiotics didn't get it all, so I had to go into the cancer center every day to get IV antibiotics. I came back to school yesterday. So far, so good.

Being home after I felt better was very difficult. It's hard to keep busy and TV gets very boring. I have a hard time reading because I can't concentrate (interferon side effect) so I actually went stir-crazy there for a while. I'm glad to be at school, where I can interact and keep myself busy.

April 2, 1998: After being back at school for a week, feeling pretty darn good, my blood test came back yesterday with a really low white count, lower hemoglobin and platelets. No wonder I don't feel as peppy as before. I go to the doctor today and we'll see what he says. I wonder what this does to my bone marrow test on Monday. I'm disappointed because I thought I might be on the upswing, but I guess not—at least at this moment in time. Life is so difficult now. It seems to be up and down, up and down—no warning—just up and down.

My life is so different. I realize now what an easy life I had before.

Now everything is such an effort: blow-drying my hair so it looks halfway decent and doesn't look so thin, socializing with people, reading (because of my concentration level), eating (because I'm never hungry). There's more, but I can't think right now.

I long for the day when I can feel better on a more consistent level—I wish I could be well again. I know I'm not the only sick person who feels this; I'm just a sick person who is experiencing these thoughts. But you can't go home again, so onward I march, however slowly.

April 8, 1998: Monday I had another bone marrow biopsy at UCLA. This time Dr. Territo did it and I didn't have to wait. She had to do it twice because she couldn't get enough for the slide, so I have more pain than usual. My white count is still low, as are my platelets and hemoglobin. Not good.

Last night I woke up so bloated I thought I would throw up. I think it was the protein drink I had in the afternoon. I took a Compazine and an Atavan to no avail. Finally I took some antacid and that did the trick. But I lost two hours of sleep.

Tonight at five thirty, I have an MRI for my ear. They put a helmet on my head so I don't move, and they'll put dye in my system. I'm quite anxious about this, but I'll get through it one way or another.

April 9, 1998: The MRI wasn't bad at all. I took two Atavans and felt relaxed—as a matter of fact, I closed my eyes and dozed a little. It took about 45 minutes total, and results come in two days.

Today I feel really good—probably the best I've felt since going on the drugs. I guess it's a good thing because open house is tonight and it will be good to feel halfway decent.

April 27, 1998: The MRI for my ear came back showing nothing. After two to three weeks of my ear being a lot better, it has clogged up again. It's very annoying.

Spring break was rather odd. It seems I struggled to find things to keep me busy. I put together the Costa Rica photo album one day, and Van and I drove out to see the poppies in Antelope Valley another day, but that was it. I don't like to be alone for a whole day. This is a new phenomenon.

3.

The Magic Bullet

It was about this time that I got a call from Virginia's dean at work who asked me to try to convince Virginia to withdraw from teaching her advanced placement course. "Van, you know Virginia's health is important to us. I think she would be much better off dropping her advanced placement class. Could you talk to her?" Virginia loved teaching that classes and her dean was trying to get me to convince her to drop it. I was disgusted and I refused. "I am not going to do that. If you want her to drop that course, you talk to her yourself." In contrast, Virginia's students were giving her lucky bamboo and anything else that would prop her up. These kids would later get the gift of seeing their compassion pay off.

I've just had a bit of a jolt. My dean called me in to talk about next year's schedule. She diplomatically told me I need to go to two preps—which means dropping my advanced placement class. I said I wanted to keep it. She said my health is more important than anything, and kids and parents have been complaining about my energy level—they're concerned about passing the A.P. test. She said it was just things she'd overheard. Yeah right. This is all very upsetting but maybe it's for the best. My dean says kids are comparing me this year to the way I was last year. At any rate, no more A.P. for me after this year.

May 12, 1998: For the past few days, I've felt a lot more energetic. It's nice to feel better for a change. Two weeks ago, our long-time friend Barbara White came down to see us. We went into June's house and had dinner and a very nice visit. Barbara gave me a full-body massage, which felt pretty good! I am able to stay up later now, so that's good, too. Dr. Blayney told me that the MRI showed a sinus infection, so I'm on antibiotics and an inhaler for a month. Interesting how the ENT never mentioned this.

My giving up the A.P. class has created quite a furor of people wanting to teach it. It's actually quite humorous. I'm glad I won't be doing that class anymore. It is really quite a relief.

I fervently hope I continue to feel better—oh, the test came back from UCLA. They tested for lymphoma instead of CML, so the whole thing was for nothing. You'd think UCLA could get it straight.

This Friday evening we have to go to the president's home for dinner with some Vietnamese dignitaries. I hope I make it OK. I'm sure I will somehow.

My one complaint health-wise now is a lump in my left side that makes me feel uncomfortable (doesn't hurt) which I've had before (last year). I thought it might be my spleen but Blayney says no. He couldn't feel it either. It's a little smaller now so hopefully it will go away.

May 21, 1998: This month has flown by. One more day and we have Memorial Day weekend. After that there are only three weeks of school left. It doesn't seem possible. I have mixed feelings. I'm glad for the "daily school routine" to come to a break, but I'm concerned about how time moves so fast. I want to be able to appreciate every moment. Sometimes the daily routine keeps me from even thinking about that.

I am still feeling better and my blood is improving. Now if the chromosome will convert, it will be a true triumph. I feel in my heart it will.

Virginia got more and more fatigued. Either the interferon or ARA-C was driving her hemoglobin down. She got so anemic that Dr. Blayney had to order transfusions. I took her to the mountains because I heard that the body responds to altitude by raising hemoglobin levels. She remembers it as a good time. I am lucky I didn't kill her. The transfusions helped, but the benefit only lasted two weeks. Each transfusion leaves a deposit of iron that builds up in the body until it can no longer tolerate transfusions. So we put off the transfusions until things got relatively bad. She had to rest every morning in order to finish drying her hair. Then the pneumonia came.

The pneumonia had been hard because it was potentially deadly, but harder for her because she had to take two weeks off from school. Thankfully Dr. Blayney knocked it back with antibiotics. Next came the spiking 104-degree fevers. Luckily we found a young infectious-disease doctor fresh out of Harvard who helped keep her going while whatever she had resolved itself. Soon afterward this doctor took a job somewhere else, but he was there when we needed him. We had moments of extraordinary fortune and this was one of them.

June 3, 1998: My wish came true! Hemoglobin is up and I do feel better. One week left of the school routine, and it's making me realize how fast time goes by. It's scary given my situation. In many ways I wish time could stand still for a while—perhaps until they have found a cure. I will make the most of my time.

One thing that I notice is how I get so many strange (actually unpleasant) smells. My hairspray drives me crazy. And there are other smells I can't even identify. I'm guessing the drugs are responsible, but who knows.

August 28, 1998: I had a rather hard start to the summer. Around June 23 or 24 I began to run a fever every day—sometimes spiking to 102. I experienced this until the end of July. I had every test imaginable, and all of them came out normal. I was under the care of an infectious disease specialist, Dr. Preston Lee. Then all of a sudden it stopped. Dr. Lee said that in 20-30 percent of cases like this, a cause is never found.

In mid-August we were able to go to Bridgeport—eighteen people came and it was a bit frustrating, but I was glad to "get out of the house." We also went to Big Bear for three days, which was nice.

It was around this time that we learned that every student in Virginia's advanced placement class had passed the national test. And so the dean needn't have worried.

All I could do was immerse myself in the topic of CML, weeding out the obvious dead ends and hoping that I was right. I did this by reading everything I could find, by pursuing every reference. I found out how to find the drugs that were in or about to go into clinical trial and read everything written about them. I found some drugs that had been tried before on other diseases and failed and were being tried again on CML. These didn't make sense to me. I found drugs that were based on concepts that just didn't make sense. It was at this time that my familiarity with CML discussion groups began to pay off.

I like discussion groups because there are always a few people grappling with the same topic I grapple with—and often at a higher level than I do. Our gem from the new discussion group was Ed Crandall, a good friend to a lot of people and especially to us. Ed had had CML for a decade, a very unusual accomplishment in those days. When Ed was diagnosed in 1980, the only proven cure for CML was a bone marrow transplant and since Ed had a donor, he decided on this course of action. He researched transplant centers and found that the Fred Hutchinson center in Washington State had the best record of success. He sold most of what he possessed and crammed the rest and his family into a Honda Civic and drove from California to Washington.

After getting his family settled into a hotel room, Ed headed to the Hutchinson Center to be prepped for the transplant. He had all the tests, the matches were good, and then it came up that Ed had had a heart attack in 1979. It wasn't long before someone showed up in the room. This person told Ed that it was unfortunate that the heart attack had not come up previously because it disqualified him from a transplant. They wished him good luck and that was it. There was Ed with his Civic, his family and the belongings that would fit inside. They all got back in the car and returned to California.

Ed went on interferon and survived the next nine years and managed to support his family as a machinist. I remember that he was a physical wreck by the time we met him. But I also remember that his mind was as sharp as a tack.

I had been reading about a line of research that involved signal transduction inhibitors. A young researcher in Oregon named Brian Druker had developed a theory that he could neutralize the BCR-ABL protein by preventing phosphorylation. He did this by attaching a small molecule to the pocket in the BCR-ABL protein where ATP attached itself and where phosphorylation occurred. With the small molecule in the way, ATP could not attach. Without phosphorylation, BCR-ABL would be turned off; and without the ability to signal and communicate reproduction and order immortality, all of them would die and the healthy cells could repopulate the marrow. Though complex, it made a lot of sense to me. I was looking for a miracle and open to something that seemed so extraordinary. Through the discussion group, Ed added his positive thought as well. He was sure he wanted to find a way into an impending trial and he thought Virginia might want to do the same. He was visiting his brother in Santa Barbara and offered to drive the 150 miles to meet with Virginia and me at an In-N-Out Burger stand in Baldwin Park that he remembered from his youth. Virginia hauled her sorry little body with me, and we met Ed. He was still driving the same Honda Civic.

At UCLA, Oregon Health and Science University, and M.D. Anderson Cancer Center in Texas, there were going to be phase 1 trials opening up for a drug designated CGP 57148B. Dr. Druker's animal studies using the drugs had been successful, and he was going to see if the drug worked the same with human beings. A phase 1 trial is officially designed as a dose-escalating trial to ascertain what doses have an effect and what doses cause harm. Most often, phase 1 trials find toxicity before they find benefit. But we were out of options. Virginia's recent bone marrow test had shown again that she had 100 percent leukemia cells, and we feared she was close to the end. Ed was so enthusiastic about this trial, and the hope in his words was palpable. Virginia left the meeting with Ed with a smile on her face. Hope again. Thank God for Ed Crandall.

By this time Virginia was off ARA-C because the doctors believed it was causing the fevers. It was surely what had caused the mouth sores. In a meeting with Dr. Blayney, he gave us the results of the last bone marrow test that we had already weaseled out of one of his staff members. He told us that the interferon was not working, which was not news to us. After he was through with his gloom and doom and clear anger over the failure, we smiled and told him that we wanted to try something else: the CGP 57148B trial. In retrospect, I think he was relieved by the conversation. He, along with most other oncologists, don't much believe in phase 1 trials, but at least he didn't have to tell Virginia to get her affairs in order. He said that he would support whatever we wanted to do. We still love that guy.

Getting into this trial was not going to be easy. We contacted Dr. Territo at UCLA and asked her to help. It happened that this was the drug that she had mentioned when we first met her. She got us an appointment with Dr. Charles Sawyers, the co-principal investigator in the UCLA branch of the phase 1 trial.

Dr. Sawyers had come to UCLA to study with Owen Witte. He had a handsome baby face and a soft manner that made you like him immediately. He was also universally described by other doctors as the smartest person any of them had ever known. Since Virginia had failed interferon, she was eligible and placed on the list of selected participants, but there were still requirements. She would have to have another bone marrow biopsy to prove the seemingly obvious fact that she had CML, and she would have to have a high white cell count of at least 20,000. Although interferon had failed to suppress the cancer, it still suppressed her counts, meaning she was going to have to end all interferon treatment to get to 20,000. On August 29, a little over a year from diagnosis, Virginia stopped the shots. There would be no turning back.

August 28, 1998: My platelets dropped so low the first week of August that Dr. Blayney took me off the ARA-C. Then my white count went so low he cut back on my interferon. This last week I went to UCLA to talk to Dr. Territo about a clinical trial. It turns out it's the drug she mentioned a year ago. Oregon, UCLA and M.D. Anderson are the only groups participating. The trial began in June, and Territo says things are promising. The drug is a tyrosine kinase inhibitor. It is aimed at eradicating a protein that is created when chromosomes 9 and 22 mix themselves up and make the leukemia cells. I have to get my white count up to 20,000 to begin participating, so I am off the drugs now, and boy do I feel good. I can eat and enjoy it, my hemoglobin is up, I have energy, my platelets are up, and it's so nice to feel better.

September 16, 1998: This is the fourth week I've been "drug free."

At the beginning of the school year (almost four weeks ago) I weighed 112; now I weigh 125. I am so pleased. It's nice to feel normal and to fit into my old clothes.

The only residual effects I have are (1) my hair is still thin and (2) my skin is still dry (but is getting better). My blood counts are normal, my hemoglobin is going up, and I feel great. Interesting thing is that my white count, which needs to be 20,000 or above to enter, is not going up very fast. In fact it's moving quite slowly: Last week it was 5.8 and this week 5.9. I guess I figured it would shoot up.

I know this may be a temporary break from controlling drugs, but I'm taking advantage of it. It's hard for me to recognize or realize I have a potentially terminal disease when I feel so great!

October 14, 1998: My blood tests are not cooperating for the clinical trial. My white count is moving up ever so slowly, my hemoglobin is normal, and my platelets are now above normal. If they go too high, I'll have to go back on the drugs. I really dread that. I know I must. When my counts stayed normal for the previous three weeks, I found myself foolishly thinking about a spontaneous remission. Oh, how wonderful that would be!

My hair is much thicker now and easier to manage. It is such a joy. My skin is less dry. My energy is high! My ear doesn't clog anymore. The only effects I still have are itching (my neck broke out into welts, and my scalp erupts into oozing patches of itching. Whether this is related to after effects or not, I don't know.

I am just going to enjoy feeling so well and do my best to maintain a positive attitude every day.

November 24, 1998: A long time has passed since I last wrote: Things have been going well. I feel great; I sense my teaching is very successful; my blood tests keep coming back normal in every way. Dr. Blayney is nervous though and says I must go back on interferon in January even if my blood is still normal. I have to be honest and say I really dread the thought of that. I'm back to my old self in all ways—I weigh 132 pounds and, have a great appetite; my hair has grown back;

I have lots of energy for aerobics three times per week and more. So it hurts to know I'll have to destroy myself again.

We are in Paris and have been seeing the sights. I took time off work with the approval of the acting principal and added it to my Thanksgiving holiday to take this trip. I never know when I can do something like this again. So I'm grabbing the opportunity while I can.

December 6, 1998: We put up the Christmas lights on the outside of the house today. I feel pretty good about this. The last day of school is December 18—two weeks. I have a lot to do between now and then. My blast counts continue to be normal. One change is that my white count seems to be on the rise. Maybe I will be able to participate in the UCLA study after all.

My life has returned to normal except for the knowledge that I have leukemia. Actually it's pretty hard for me to believe most of the time. I relish feeling energetic and having all my hair. I so enjoy going to aerobics three times per week; it makes me feel so normal. I thank God for this reprieve and I pray something big will happen.

I look forward to Christmas and being able to do what I have always done.

December 26, 1998: Well, what a wonderful Christmas Day! I so enjoyed having everyone for dinner and feeling energetic. As a matter of fact, at the end of the day, my feet hurt because I'd been on them all day!

We got the best Xmas present ever Monday, December 21. At UCLA we met Dr. Sawyers, the head of the tyrosine kinase inhibitor clinical trial, who turned out to be a very nice man. He told us I was a good candidate for the study, and he could hardly contain his excitement at how successfully the drug is working. He also told us that the report we read is outdated and that the results are even better now; reading between the lines, the results go way beyond the 80 percent success rate. Dr. Sawyers also said that my CML is young, as indicated by my quick return to normal of my white count when I began treatment. That was nice to hear. When we left UCLA, Connie, Van, and I were walking on clouds. I can begin probably in late January or early February when my white count goes above 20,000. Dr. Sawyers will call Dr. Blayney to tell him not to put me back on interferon. For all these things, I am so very grateful.

The period between stopping interferon and starting the inhibitor was a lot longer than anticipated. Virginia had blood tests at Pomona Valley Hospital every week, but the effects of interferon lingered and at first the white counts didn't move. Then they began to move up, but slowly. All this time the trial was progressing. Ed stopped his interferon and got in early at 25 mg of the drug. There was no response, but he was still hopeful. At each center the trial would progress on with cohorts of two patients entering the trial, each on a higher dose than the two before. Then, with great sorrow to us, Ed Crandall died. He had started the trial at a dose that was too low to save him. The last time I talked to him he was very ill. He had been offered a dose that might have saved him, but he just could not. I offered him a room at Cal Poly and a ride in to UCLA, but it was too late. He died two days later. Still, Virginia and I were committed and had to proceed. We still grieve for Ed.

Virginia began to feel better almost immediately as the interferon began to dissipate and her white blood count got to 10,000 but she needed to reach 20,000. The trial dose was up to 140 mg. Still, there was no clinical benefit. The trial got to 200 mg and still no response from anyone. Virginia felt great by this time. Her white count was at 15,000, above normal, but still too low to start. A nurse told us that if Virginia ran up and down the stairs before having a blood test, the counts might be higher. Silly as this sounds, we did it. Then, as the trial dose reached 300 mg, Virginia reached 20,000. She got through a final physical and was scheduled to start at a dose of 350 mg. Rumors flowed through the discussion group that researchers had seen results at 300.

January 6, 1999: I don't quite know how to express myself on this subject. I feel left out of the loop on so many things at work. Sometimes I feel bad about things coming to this, but I guess that's life. It has also started to bother me how I imagine people talking about me behind my back. I feel like everyone is "treading softly" so as not to offend/bother me, etc.

I realize these are not worthy of my emotional reactions, but feelings are facts.

January 30, 1999: My white count is still hovering just above normal. Last week it went down to 10,000; this week it is 12.4 or so. Van got very nervous, so he called Dr. Blayney as well as Dr. Sawyers at UCLA. Sawyers said, "DON'T WORRY! This is good! It means she had a strong positive reaction to the interferon." So we are just waiting and enjoying! Dr. Sawyers said they know who I am and I'm on the list, and they may be opening up the study to more people—even people below 20,000 white count—sooner than they thought. So life is good.

February 12, 1999: My skin continues to blotch up on my neck with redness and then dries up to flaky patches. Tonight my scalp did its weepy thing, too—first time in a long time. Guess I'd better go to a dermatologist.

My white count went up to 13.9 this week. Maybe I'm on my way to UCLA.

February 20, 1999: It is a lovely day and I'm sitting on the back patio appreciating the beautiful backyard. My impatiens are all gone due to frost about a month ago, but the camellias are blooming and the grass and shrubs are a lovely green. There is a slight chill in the air after a warm day in the 70s.

It is hard for me to believe I have this life-threatening disease and even harder to believe I could die from it. Once in a while, I try to imagine my house, my things, my dogs, my husband without me. It is almost impossible. Something in me won't allow that speculation to continue for too long. I do wonder what Van would do with my things. How would he get along? I would hope he would find someone else to help him "walk life's path," but I'm not willing to abdicate my position yet.

My blood count was up again this week to 14.1. I'm on my way to UCLA. I know this new drug is the answer, and I can't wait to participate and receive its benefits.

My mind more often now strays to counterproductive thought of how did this happen to me? What caused it? I think back on the birth control pills I took, the pesticide they sprayed in New Jersey and Hemet, where I grew up, the food I've eaten from the microwave, the whitener I used on my teeth, the sunless tanning lotion I used, and anything else that comes to my mind, and I wonder, "Was that it?" Then I realize how many other people have been exposed to the same things and don't have leukemia and I drop it. Is it that my genes are defective? I hate to feel as if I'm defective. I've tried so hard to do the things to make me healthy and vigorous, which is why it seems so unfair.

But what is, is. And I must deal with what is aggressively and without fear. Life has been good to me. Now it's my turn to give life all I've got. To do less is unacceptable to me. And so we beat on, boats against the current.

February 24, 1999: A couple days ago we attended the funeral of Eleanor Farrand's mother. It was held in the Episcopal Church in San Gabriel on the San Marino line. When we were entering the church (late), they were singing "Holy, Holy, Holy." I found to my amazement that I knew all the verses by heart—after how many years!? When the liturgy called for reciting the twenty-third psalm, I remembered how many times I had said that lonely verse to myself last year—every bone marrow biopsy—times when I felt very ill—during my MRI, Gallium scan, heart test. It was comforting, so soothing. I never thought I'd need something like that, and I'm so glad I had it at my disposal.

February 28, 1999: Last day of February! A lovely one, too. We went to Prado Regional Park to see if the boat Van and the boys built would float. It did just fine. It's a pretty boat and it works just like a boat should. The day is warm, sunny, and a bit breezy—the kind of day that makes one realize winter is ending and spring is promised. My sweet peas are eight inches high and I'll need to put up a net within the week. It will be nice to have sweet-smelling flowers this spring. Again, my joy in these small things seems to contradict my stage of life due to my disease. It is so hard to realize I'm sick. I feel so good; I'm strong; I enjoy working out—including boxing every Tuesday night—to look at me, you would think I'm excruciatingly healthy. Life is good.

March 12, 1999: It struck me today that it is sad that I got new carpeting and drapes for the house and never really got to enjoy them the first year because I was sick. The carpet in the living room is fairly ruined with Bonnie's pooping and peeing. It's a real shame, but not to be helped. I've had my little fur child since she was a puppy and now she is so old and infirm.

March 14, 1999: Went to nephew Craig's baseball game yesterday. I had my hat and sunglasses on but I still broke out with itchy welts on my face and neck—even on the back of my neck. Who knows why this happens.

Today I worked in the yard a bit. Planted some shasta daisies in the bed by the carport. Sweet peas are growing nicely up the net. They should be lovely when they bloom. This is the time of year when all growing things seem so promising. The birds sing happily, the buds bud, and I love it. How nice to be able to enjoy it this year.

I really like my house, my neighborhood, my town, my hair, my hairdresser, my dog groomer, my pharmacy, my donut shop, my oncologist, my oncologist nurses, my UCLA doctors, my car, my cleaners/laundry, etc.

March 29, 1999: It was fun to go to Mt. Sac to watch my nephew Stephen's swim meet. Many area high schools were there, including DBHS with several kids I know on the team—especially Jeremy Tomista in my first period English II class. Stephen is quite a swimmer and has quite a buff body. Looks just like swimmers do.

My white count was 17.4 last week but my platelets broke 800(000). Who knows what will happen? Bad news tonight is making me both sad and nervous and edgy. Ed Crandall, the man we met last summer who was in the UCLA program (kicked out because the low dosage didn't control his white count), is in blast crisis and doesn't have long to live. His daughter relayed this via an e-mail. This reminds me that my time is indeed finite—this could happen to me at any moment. It is strange how I can calmly ponder and write about this. Is it because I don't really believe it will happen? At any rate, it is very sad to be aware of and be powerless to help. The same feeling as I have about my disease. How long will I continue to do well? Will I be saved? Will UCLA do it for me?

Will I have to go back on interferon? If so, how long will that give me? When I allow myself to think of these things, I become angry—and that is counterproductive.

Tomorrow, Mother has her second cataract removed. I hope all goes well. I'll be praying.

April 2, 1999: Unfortunately, on Tuesday I found out Shirley Shuler's daughter-in-law who had a BMT at City of Hope and who had very bad bouts with graft-host disease but who overcame everything and went home, died. She left behind three little kids and a husband. This would be so devastating. In addition to this, Lance Gross told me Lindsey, who had a BMT last year at City of Hope, is having a bout with graft-host disease after several months of being fine and has to go back on medication.

My white count is 18.2 this week and my platelets are slightly lower. All is well.

Today begins spring break. I got all my work done at school, so I'm fine! It will be a fun time.

April 6, 1999: Mother's birthday—she's eighty-one years old (and doing very well indeed). We're going out to take her to lunch and celebrate.

News flash! My blood count is up to 20.4, and I can now get into the UCLA study. Van called today. They said it might be two weeks or it could be this Friday if a person who is waiting for his white count to go up doesn't make it to 20,000. All of a sudden life is uncertain again. Unsettled I am, wondering I am, worrying I am. Will this drug work? Will it make me sick? What will happen? I am reminded I am indeed diseased and I need to have a very close relationship with my medical professional to get myself out of this. I still know in my heart I will get out of this and I will triumph. "I am stronger than you are; you cannot defeat me."

I was thinking back on last summer when I was at my all-time low. I'm particularly reminded of the sinus infection that caused me to blow blood and blood clots out my nose. I just dealt with it because I had no choice. It was truly an alarming thing. I think I was using a box of Kleenex every two days. Also dry mouth and parched, chapped lips. I'd be getting up every hour at night for a drink of water so my throat wouldn't stick together. Praying my temperature wouldn't go up/ that I wouldn't have to go into the hospital/that I wouldn't get pneumonia again. It was really a terrible time, but I gained more time out of it—it was well worth it. I'd like to think it's over.

I've been religiously attending aerobics classes three times per week. Club boxing required me to purchase my own boxing gloves. I love to punch the punching bags. Kick-boxing is fun, too. I hope this will be good for me in the future.

April 8, 1999: I'm grateful for......

A husband who gives me unlimited love and support.

My energy.

My sweet little dog's health.

My thick hair.

My mother's health.

Got a call from Ginny Naessig, the clinical research coordinator for the UCLA study. It looks like I might be able to begin April 27 and be part of the next "cohort" (dosing group).

Regarding what she said...

Days before I have a bone marrow biopsy—can do it here with Blayney, an EKG.

Various blood labs.

I go in for twenty-six hours. Blood is drawn every hour almost. I stay in the clinic, not the actual hospital.

I have blood tests every Monday and Thursday or every Tuesday and Friday.

I see Dr. Sawyers once a week for the first twenty-eight days.

At the end of twenty-eight days, I go in for twenty-four hours and have a bone marrow biopsy.

Then go on next twenty-eight days.

They are at 350 mg now—will go to 400 in next cohort (maybe me). Have plans to go to 475 then 550, maybe higher if no side effects.

Side Effects:

Mild GI upset that Mylanta took care of in two people.

One person with liver function problem—off drug for a week, returned to normal (M.D. Anderson).

Tingling in feet for one person.

The bleeding ulcer the guy already had got aggravated.

One person who came in was at a 60,000 white count—the drug is bringing it down.

Typically white count goes up for first week, and then comes down. They are having great success with the white counts being controlled. So far, though no PH chromosome conversions, although one man who's been on the drug for six months hasn't had a bone marrow biopsy recently and Ginny Naessig says he'll have one soon. Perhaps when people have been on the high doses for months they will see conversion.

April 16, 1999: Very busy week! Monday I got home and got a call from Ginny Naessig. She said there was an opening now and I need to get some tests—bone marrow biopsy, blood work, pregnancy test, EKG. And so began a challenging odyssey.

Tuesday—bone marrow biopsy at 9:30 a.m. at Dr. Blayney's because he leaves at ten for airport. Connie comes, and so does Van. I go to school and teach first period—get coverage for second and third and go for test.

I return to school after the painful ordeal of these tests.

At the junction of Interstates 10 and 57, I feel wetness on my back. It is blood seeping out of the bandage onto my clothes and the seat.

I decide to apply pressure and continue on to work. My arm and hand are in an obtuse position that is extremely uncomfortable. I make it to school and walk to the nurse's office where I call Wilshire Oncology after I see how much I'm bleeding. When I got into the bathroom to take off blood-soaked underpants and pants, I saw the blood dripping onto the floor.

I lie down and apply pressure as told to do by Helen at the doctor's for fifteen minutes. I am in a very uncomfortable position.

Bleeding stops, and I limp to class for fear of disturbing wound and bringing on more bleeding. Stacy Lund leaves and I stay, not sitting down.

In fifteen minutes, it bleeds once more. I get Stacy and leave to drive back to Wilshire Oncology, where I lie down on my stomach with three IV bags tied together and Vickie's hand applying pressure on the wound.

Forty minutes later, it stops bleeding and I get a pressure bandage with very tight adhesive tape. I turn over, and lie on a pillow on my back for fifteen more minutes.

I get up and am told to walk around, sit, etc., to see how it "holds." I'm OK and I go back to sixth period.

My heart starts to skip beats and I have to go for an EKG after school. I go, register at the cardio respiratory department, and have the EKG. My heart skips a couple of times. The woman who does the test tells me her sister is in the City of Hope with acute leukemia, losing her hair and doing very poorly. Our birthdays are two days apart.

Wednesday—Van bird-dogs test results and faxes them to UCLA. At two fifteen he calls and says Pomona Valley lost my EKG. I rush out of school, leaving instructions for a sub (since I'm going to UCLA the next day) and have another EKG before I go to my 3:20 p.m. appointment at the dentist. I'm glad my heart "behaved."

When I returned home from the dentist, Van told me my EKG came back abnormal, with the note, "can't rule out an infarction at an unspecified date."

Ginny tells me my appointment for induction into the program is Monday, April 19 at eleven forty-five. The EKG won't keep me out of the program.

She further tells me they had the first person whose chromosomes converted—50 percent—yea!

On April 19, 1999 we had our meeting with Dr. Sawyers to start the trial. My sister, a steady support to us both, came along. Dr. Sawyers confirmed that they had seen significant clinical benefit at 300 mg. He handed Virginia her first dose of the drug—350 mg—and after a nervous amount of chatter that was driving me mad, she was finally nudged into taking them. Virginia says we all leaned forward to see if her arms would fall off or if something equally awful would happen. Of course, nothing awful did happen. It seemed an anticlimactic end to a long and nervous eight months, but I assure you that the three of us left with big smiles hiding massive emotions. We were on our way to a miracle.

April 19, 1999: UCLA day! The first time I take the drug. It is a momentous occasion as I hold the drug in my hand and chat with Ginny the nurse. Van says, "Come on already—swallow it!" Van's sweet sister Connie is there too...my heart pounds...I wait after I swallow the pills, 350 mg of CGP57148B, as if expecting something monumental to happen. Nothing does. All goes well and I'm on the road.

In those days, you were not encouraged to fraternize with your fellow trial participants. We learned later that I knew her partner at 350 mg. David Lawyer was a teacher in Santa Barbara and one who had been teaching at UCSB when I was in graduate school.

Connie, Virginia, and I left UCLA happy and hopeful and headed straight to McDonald's for a Big Mac. This became our tradition. To supplement our serious research, we were covering our bases with good old American superstition. We continued to frequent McDonald's for good luck; we collected lucky coins off the street; and every time we found a temple in Asia or a church where we could, we lit incense or candles.

Although interferon didn't show any sign of saving Virginia in the long run, we think it gave her the year she needed to wait for a medical breakthrough. It turned out that 300 mg was the threshold for the drug to be effective, and she and the remainder of the cohort got 350 mg two weeks later. This meant that she was one of the first few people to receive an effective dose. We had to wait to see if it would work for her.

Admittedly the people who took this drug were all desperate to find a way to live—to see wives, husbands, children and grandchildren grow up, but in my book, they are also heroes. They stepped into the unknown and helped demonstrate that Brian Druker was right. He had found a way to control chronic myelogenous leukemia. Ed Crandall gave his life while helping to save Virginia and all the others who would contract CML in the future.

Based on the sacrifice of a friend and the courage of Virginia and the others who participated in the phase 1 trial, we had new hope and we didn't dwell on the sadness; we had to look ahead. We were now living in the world of tyrosine kinase inhibitors. We were in a trial that could turn south at any time. Virginia was alive and feeling good, but the black hole we had been looking at was still there because ours was still the world of the unknown.

A good friend, psychologist and cancer survivor, Barbara White, once told us that of the cancer survivors she counseled, all of them, no matter what they had gone through, said they would not want to give up the ordeal. These people had learned so much from the experience and the transformation it had caused in them that they never wanted to go back. Eventually, we too began to take some stock of what we had learned and become through the experience, and we were ready to move on.

4.

Bullseye

The trial's tyrosine kinase inhibitor, CGP57148B, was soon renamed STI 571 and although it seemed to be working for all those involved, for us there was still a level of high anxiety. Would this wonder continue? On the face of things, CML had one line of communication. STI 571 blocked that line of communication, thereby weakening the disease, and possibly exterminating it. But what if the protein found a way around the drug and signaled through another pathway? How would Virginia or any of the others react to the drug? Would this last? Would the drug company keep producing it?

May 10, 1999: I'm in the waiting room at UCLA oncology center waiting for my weekly check-in. I thought my heart was getting a little better, but it sure is doing flip flops now. Time will tell.

Last week a little girl in my first-period class, Cynthia Mercado, ran (literally) up to me in the library while I was in line to turn in tests (SAT 9) and asked me in her sweet little voice, "Mrs. Garner, do you have cancer?"

"Yes Cynthia, I have leukemia, a cancer of the blood."

"Oh Mrs. Garner, I'm going to pray for you every day."

Cynthia is one of my special ed. kids and a very sweet little girl.

I am touched by so many things my kids do. Every day at 8:45 a.m., one of the kids or another reminds me to take my pills. Usually I need the reminder. They are so concerned.

May 12, 1999: Yesterday, Jackie Erlansan called to find out how I was doing. Her husband had a perfect match—very rare in an unrelated donor, so they did some research on the Internet from Hutchinson Center in Seattle and found out that since he had a perfect match and is in his late thirties, he has almost an 80 percent chance of total success. He decided to go for it. So the transplant is scheduled for July.

They talked to their City of Hope doctor about my drug, and they said it was a very unsure thing because it has not been tested. I wonder now—did I make the right decision? Should I have gone for the BMT? The chances are only 30 to 60 percent because of my age. I've cut myself off now due to the fact you have to do it in the first year for maximum effectiveness. Have I sealed my fate? Have I precluded the possibility of chromosome conversion on interferon by switching to this new drug? These things come to the front of my mind at times. But I know I mustn't dwell on them.

I'm confident the drug I'm taking will be the answer.

Last week the USB kids came trooping into my room during fourth period with a bouquet of flowers, a sweatshirt, a towel, and a bunch of purple and gold balloons. I had been dubbed Renaissance Teacher of the Month. Kids from my classes had voted for me in the USB room. It was a thrill! Virginia is back!!!

May 25, 1999: Last Monday I was released on my own recognizance for a month. I don't have to go to UCLA until June 14. On that day I have a bone marrow biopsy. This I can wait for! Things are going very well. I admit I sometimes think about "the road not taken," but I can't waste too much effort on that. When I think back on a year ago and how anemic I was and what the end of the year was like, I thank God how wonderful it is this year. Things couldn't be better.

Five things I'm grateful for!

My feeling good.

My mother's health.

Bonnie's health.

Van's support.

The sweet kids I have at school.

Virginia's mind was clearing and she felt great. She looked healthy, but we still had no evidence that the drug was working to eliminate the disease. In June 1999, she had her fifth bone marrow biopsy, the second for the study. In two weeks, we got the results—no change, still 100 percent leukemia cells. Soon Virginia's white counts began to drop precipitously. You need white cells, and in particular neutrophils, to fight off infections. The doctors didn't know what to do. You cannot transfuse white cells. There are drugs, Neupogen and Leukine primarily, that stimulate the marrow to produce more white blood cells, but giving them was not written into the trial protocol so Dr. Sawyers would have had to ask for a change to do it. He couldn't have presented a very strong case since no one knew if the stimulants might also accelerate the development of cancer cells. According to protocol, at an absolute neutrophil count (ANC) of 1.5, Dr. Sawyers temporarily pulled Virginia off the drug. We were again looking at the black hole. Five days later she was back on the drug. Two days later she was off. Five days later she was back on. This was the pattern for more than a month until August, when the magic number in the protocol was changed from 1.5 to a lower 1, meaning she could stay on the drug longer. Still, a less radical form of cycling continued. What worried us was that while Virginia was cycling off and on the drug, as far as we knew, most of the other patients had no trouble. Blood tests began twice a week and then only once. Luckily, Virginia has good veins. I remember once or twice when the blood tests at Wilshire Oncology showed an ANC of less than 1, I drove her to UCLA for another test because they generally read higher there. It seems a bit humorous now, but we were desperate for her to stay on the drug.

June 13, 1999: School's over. Graduation was June tenth. It was sad to say goodbye to my kids this year. We have been on quite a journey together. But the minutes, hours, days, weeks, months, and years just keep "movin on." I do so wish I could stop time.

On Wednesday, June 2, a small glitch happened in my progress in the UCLA study. Ginny Naessig called me at school to tell me my absolute neutrophil count went below 1.5 (it was 1.3) and they were pulling me off the drug until it returned to a number above 1.5. Ever since it has gone down. Today is the eleventh day off the drug. I had a blood test last week— Monday through Friday. Pomona Valley Hospital always gives low readings compared to UCLA, so Van wants me to go to

UCLA to corroborate. It's always higher there. Friday, Pomona said it was .7 and UCLA said it was 1.2.

Monday, tomorrow, I go back to UCLA to have a bone marrow biopsy. I cringe at the thought of the pain and I'm afraid of bleeding again. I pray there's some PH+ chromosome conversion, and I'm worried that being off the drug may jeopardize that. I yearn to walk into the light.

June 30, 1999: Since the last entry, I've been on the drug for two days—white count got down again—off for five days—on again at reduced dosage of 300 mg (originally it was 350), white count went from 1.8 to 1.7 in three days—we'll see. Peripheral blood from bone marrow shows no chromosome conversion. Disappointing, but I really had been on the drug for only two months. Still I have to fight feeling disheartened. What if I made a bad decision? What if this drug doesn't work on me like it does on other people? Why is this happening to me? I spend so much of my time feeling "normal" now because I feel so good; then the shadow of this killer disease hovers over me and I'm filled with the reality that I'm not normal at all! Actually people are very kind to me in remarking how good I look, but I'm tired of the subscript: "You look so good—you don't look like you're going to die." I feel bad for feeling like that, too. It doesn't seem right, but as my old principal Walt Holmes said, "Feelings are facts."

Two days from now, I'm supposed to go to China and Vietnam with Van. With my blood count so unstable, I must have blood tests when we are in Hong Kong. The logistics of it are driving me into a full-blown anxiety attack.

—Will they accept the prescription for the tests?

—Will they fax it to UCLA?

—Will I be able to communicate with Ginny? Every time I call, her answering machine is on.

—Will my blood go too low again?

—If so, will I "catch" something awful?

I realize this is neurotic behavior on my part, but I'm helpless to control it. Actually I've lost the sense of controlling anything in my life.

It occurs to me that we all labor under the false assumption that we do have control of our lives. We think if we eat the right things, exercise, live good lives, we won't fall ill—we will prevent heart disease, cancer, stroke, etc. We think if we drive safely, we won't be killed or maimed on the highway. I guess I'm proof that we really don't have control of anything.

Virginia was still feeling well, and we did our best to adjust our outlooks and also to lead a normal life. I still needed to keep my job, and part of it entailed international travel. Virginia had traveled with me in the past, and in July she started to travel again. The challenge was getting blood tests overseas. I remember the sweetest little nun in Hong Kong's Matilda Hospital who drew Virginia's blood. Fifteen minutes and twenty-five dollars later, we had the results. The ANC was over 1. An ANC of more than 1 was a bargain at any price. She promised to send the results to UCLA and she did.

July 9: Taxi in the fog to the top of "the peak" to have a blood test at the Matilda Hospital. Paid for by credit card! Needle and syringe in package—syringe emptied into collection vial—not directly filled as in USA. Very nice people. Faxed results to UCLA. So far I've heard nothing, so I assume all is well.

I am thankful for:

Being able to travel once again and learn new things.

Feeling good every day.

My family—Van, Mother, Don and Sammy, the boys and Connie and Frank.

Our neighbors Karen and Bud McAndrew.

Being able to work out in my yard.

In Vietnam we worried more about finding a clean place to get Virginia tested, but we found an international medical clinic. We went into the office, put our name on a list and sat down in the waiting room. Soon, a young Australian doctor came wandering out among the patients looking for the sick leukemia patient. He couldn't find her and soon called out Virginia's name. She did look terrific. He was astounded. We explained the new drug and the importance of the blood tests. The results were again above 1. We were good again for the drug. I wish we could have had a drink with that doctor who shared our feeling of victory. I like to think he had a drink for us and then went on to have a wonderful and prosperous practice somewhere. We knew something was going right.

July 13, 1999: Hanoi. Most interesting experience—going to AEA (don't ask me what the letters stand for) to get blood test.

Walk in, very gleaming, white, clean. Explain why we're there. Give letter and prescription to receptionist who speaks some English. She takes the info and disappears. My heart beats fast and hard. The next thing...

Dr. Tim Moore from Australia appears, calling my name and surprising me. He tells me he didn't expect Virginia Garner to be me because I look so good! I explain about the study I'm in, and he seems impressed.

Blood drawn in a very hygienic room by very hygienic technician. She draws blood directly into vial and asks me if I need to lie down. She says the French always need to lie down. Ha!

We pay for tests—$26—and walk back to hotel on busy streets of Hanoi. I am so relieved. Van buys me a bouquet of roses from a cute Vietnamese lady.

We were becoming quite the celebrities at UCLA thanks to these blood tests from exotic places.

Virginia's ANC plummeted again, but we discovered that the automated machines were unable to read Virginia's counts correctly. After we switched to a manual count, Virginia's true ANC was found to be much higher than was previously thought. With the changed ANC rules and after changing over to manual counts, Virginia was able to stay on the drug longer.

When more patients started getting STI 571, it became clear that the drop in white counts was more common than the doctors had thought it would be. The cancerous white cells were being killed faster than the few remaining healthy cells could repopulate the body. The drop in ANC, and more important the stabilization of counts, meant that something good was going on.

August 23, 1999: At UCLA. Saw Dr. Sawyers and Ginny. Big shock—a person came into the waiting room at seven thirty and asked for me. I asked if there was a problem and she said my ANC was .4! Needed to know my doctor's name so she could immediately page him. He didn't act worried when he saw me and looked at the smear. He said that by eyeballing it, it seemed to be above 1, enough to keep on the drug. But I had another blood draw, and it said just above 1—OK to continue on the drug. They don't want me off. (I don't want to go off either) but my ANC is low, just over 1, the cutoff.

Dr. Sawyers had said 50 to 60 percent of those in blast crisis get out of the crisis, but now it looks like they (some of them) relapse while on the drug—meaning the cells find some way around it—the first ominous news about this drug. Back to my original question—what will become of me? Will Novartis continue this research or ditch this drug? Will I go back to interferon? Get so sick again? Lose the hair I've finally regrown? Will I die from this disease? I refuse to think of anything besides my success. I know I will succeed.

September 6, 1999: School starts tomorrow. I'm excited to be able to "do my thing" without physical challenges. I can't help thinking about my predicament. I know what the inevitable is, and I resist that reality. Talked to Brad Erlanson who had the BMT in July and he's doing well. He weathered some tough times but is cancer free and feels pretty good. Did I make the right decision? Have I with that decision sealed my fate? I couldn't help but envy Brad.

I'm nervous about the bone marrow test that looms before me and the possibility that the results will not be any better than last time. What will happen if this is the case?

On September 20, 1999, Virginia got her third bone marrow biopsy from the study. Two weeks later, we learned what we thought we already knew. The drug was working. She had 20 percent normal cells. We were beyond happy. Virginia was feeling well, and she had joined her fellow patients on the success side of the program.

October 3, 1999: Went in for bone marrow biopsy September 20. Highlights of the last month:

—Smooth beginning of school.

—Telling new kids about my appointment @UCLA and why I had it.

—Telling a "fellow" he would not be doing my BMB.

—Dr. Sawyers saying the longer people are on the drug, the better they do.

—Waiting for results—preparing myself for no change.

—Hemoglobin also below normal.

—Thursday, September 30: getting news from Ginny at UCLA that my white cells were only 80 percent PH+—20 percent NORMAL!! Glory Hallelujah!

—Being swept up in a tide of joy—sheer joy—tempered with the knowledge that things can change so quickly!

Life is so good at moments like this. It's a feeling I didn't know about until this happened to me. I feel blessed.

Sometimes true miracles happen. This is one of those times.

I'm thankful for:

Feeling good every day.

Having hair.

Bonnie bouncing back from her crisis in August and chomping dry dog food and feeling pretty good.

My mother's health.

My eternal support, Van.

Connie, who is behind me 100 percent no matter what.

In fact, the three centers conducting the study were now seeing a great deal of success. Almost every patient who was getting STI 571 at a level of 300 mg or more was seeing cancer loads diminish. And most patients, including Virginia, were once again experiencing health and vitality that had been impossible under interferon. In early October, Virginia received a call from UCLA asking her if she would mind talking to people from CNN. Not only were we excited that Virginia might be on CNN, but it also indicated that UCLA considered her a success. It meant that of all the patients at UCLA, they viewed Virginia as the one they wanted to showcase. Maybe we had won. Maybe.

What followed was a heady time. The CNN team interviewed and videoed Virginia at home and at work. I think her students realized what their support had meant. It seemed that they had participated in a miracle, and they were on TV as well. Dr. Blayney and Dr. Sawyers were interviewed too. It bonded us more closely to our doctors than ever. With all our friends, we watched the television and there Virginia was, talking about the miracle of this new drug and that it was a possible paradigm shift in the treatment of cancer. We got calls from friends in other countries who saw the piece. Virginia found herself quoted in dozens of newspapers across the country. Friends called to let her know that they shared her joy. People she didn't know, those she'd given hope to, called as well.

October 24, 1999: Big-time news! I'll be on CNN tomorrow. Dr. Sawyers is making an announcement at a press conference tomorrow morning and UCLA had reporters calling to interview some patients. Ginny called to ask me because she thought of me immediately. So Friday, Mark, a reporter, and Jeff, a photographer, came and interviewed me at home. They took shots of me in the backyard with my dogs and in the dining room with me correcting papers, and in the kitchen where I showed them my pills and talked about them. We'll see if I appear to be a complete idiot!

This development is sooo significant because it means they are confident enough to announce publicly what's going on. May all this continue. Mazel tov!

November 7, 1999: The CNN segment was very nice. It's 2:55 long and I'm on it for about fifteen seconds. First I'm in the kitchen showing the drug I call "precious pills," then I'm in an interview saying people will be amazed at this new drug. Then I'm in the backyard with fur children Bonnie and Annie. The story was very accurate and informative. I was pleased.

My life is so normal now that when it registers that I still have a potentially fatal disease it shoots stabs of fear through me. I had a dream last night that UCLA called me in to tell me the drug company had decided to stop producing STI 571 due to lack of effectiveness—or they didn't think it would be cost effective. They were letting me know that once the supply is depleted, there will be no more drug. My hope for survival was dashed, and then I woke up.

November 14, 1999: I am feeling bad that my disease has been so hard for Van. One of Van's colleagues told me Van stood in the entry hall of Kellogg House last week and said, "I feel like two years of darkness have just lifted."

I am thankful for:

Van feeling better about life.

Me feeling so healthy and looking pretty good.

My Bonnie being so spunky and healthy.

In November, CNN interviewed Virginia again in preparation for the announcements of STI 571's success at the December 1999, American Society of Hematology Conference. Again, Virginia, along with others, was an articulate, vibrant, and grateful representative of the program. She was on CNN again and then on NBC. I thought it was fun, but the critical thing was that it made Virginia important to the trial in a way others might not be. In retrospect, I believe that if Virginia had been more anonymous, she would have received the same treatment, but then I was not sure.

November 21, 1999: Tomorrow CNN comes to film me at school with a class and walking into school, etc. Big hullabaloo at the district office. Ginny Naessig never called me back regarding my concern as to whether this was OK—so I'm going ahead with it. I certainly don't want to upset UCLA, but I don't know what to do. December is a big report at the ASH conference so time will tell what happens. All this makes me nervous. I don't want to jinx the success I (and others) have had so far.

November 27, 1999: Wow! So much has happened since I last wrote. The CNN taping went well, the only problem being that the idiot public relations person from our district insisted that a reporter and photographer from the Daily Bulletin attend. I felt sorry for the CNN photographers, and it made me angry that this man would be so presumptuous.

On Monday, November 29 at 5 p.m., CNN will tape Dr. Sawyers and me at UCLA—what a trip!! This story is to air on December 5 at 3 p.m. or later. I find myself becoming more and more uneasy, especially as my five-month bone marrow biopsy approaches (December 20). Of course I ask myself, will the wonderful effects of this drug last! I pray they will. I do, however, feel uneasy.

December 18, 1999: I was on CNN again on December 3. It was supposed to air December 5, but ABC jumped the gun. This time, it was connected to the ASH (American Society of Hematologists) Conference. Dr. Druker (head investigator) of Oregon Health Center announced the results of the phase 1 trial as astounding and very unexpected—that people responded so well. It makes me nervous even though I'm very happy. I'm so grateful for this time of well-being and hope.

January 7, 2000: "It is a lucky world"—a quote by a five-year-old girl who had a five-organ transplant and survived. I would have to concur. The century/millennium rolled over with little fanfare here. Van and I nested in and watched TV coverage. January 1, 2000 was spent watching the Rose Parade, watching Craig fishing at Prado, and watching the Rose Bowl and Cotton Bowl games.

On February 28, the Chicago Tribune reported, "When future historians look back, they may well divide the nation's protracted War on Cancer into the years before and after STI 571."

In spite of all this enthusiasm for the experimental drug keeping Virginia alive, it soon became clear that there was serious doubt about whether Novartis would continue the development of the drug. We had underestimated the possibility that a pharmaceutical company might pull the plug. Company planners authorized the trial without anticipating its great success. They had been willing to produce a few kilos of STI 571, which would be enough for the people who would be accepted into the trial and who it was presumed would also likely die before they had a need for more. But almost everyone had survived, everyone needed more of the drug, and there wasn't enough. There was a real chance that the company would drop a drug that could save the relatively few numbers of people who needed it since the investment needed to proceed would not reap a high profit. During the time Virginia went off and on her drug because of the low ANC, she had accumulated a stash of extra drug. During this time, we protected it like gold.

Peter Rowbotham, whose wife Rita had CML and was in the study, and a talented young woman, Susan McNamara, who had CML, worked together to craft wording for an Internet petition that asked Novartis to scale up the production of its drug and to continue into phase 2 trials. Four thousand people signed the petition that was hand-delivered by Susan to Novartis in Switzerland. Lucky for all CML patients, the plea landed on the desk of a man of character, Novartis CEO Daniel Vasella, who as a physician, realized the importance of what was happening and personally ordered the production of twenty tons of the drug. Still, the company struggled to keep trials supplied while new production facilities were being constructed. It was possible that there would be more patients on STI 571 than anyone had ever anticipated. In the end Novartis benefited financially from Chairman Vasella's ethical decision.

While Virginia was settling into her role as celebrity queen and enjoying her feeling of health and hope, and the CML discussion group was exercising its power, I couldn't help but worry that the fairy tale would collapse on us. I dug into my research. I learned a number of tricks that helped me eliminate topics that would waste time, but I still read from the time I got home from work to two and three in the morning. With STI 571 in my life, it should have become easier, but there were new problems to consider. In December, 1999, Virginia got her fourth bone marrow biopsy through the study. Even with cycling on and off, she now had 60 percent normal cells; any problems with her white cells had passed, but not everything was perfect. Her tests showed something called a 12/12 translocation. My research seemed to show it to be of no concern, but it was to me anyway. It was also obvious that the drug was suppressing other blood counts, in particular platelets (thrombocytopenia) and hemoglobin (anemia). The platelet counts got so low that the trial protocol required her to start cycling on and off again, but Virginia's optimism overrode most negative thoughts.

January 21, 2000: My December 20 bone marrow test came back

60 percent normal cells! This STI 571 really is working. I pray its effects will be sustained.

March 5, 2000: Yesterday I sent an email to Brian Druker to thank him for my life. He answered me within an hour. That's so impressive. He said, "I don't know about this hero thing [I called him my hero], but I am trying to adapt." Typical humility.

March 19, 2000: March is almost over and I can't believe how swiftly the days have passed. Actually, it is frightening to me. My illness has focused the idea that time is so precious and I seem to have one foot in my normal mode of appreciating each day, each moment. Anything can happen at any time—actually it's that way for everyone, not just those of us who are living with life-threatening diseases. But, I go for days forgetting that this is so, taking my 300 mg of STI 571 as if the pills were vitamins. What a miracle it would be if this were to be the way I live for the next twenty to thirty years or even more!

Tomorrow I go to UCLA for another bone marrow test. I think about it with not only anxiety about the pain I know I'll have, but with nervous anticipation of the results. Will my PH+ cells be more or less? Will the 12/12 translocation still be there? Will it be more? Less? I know for sure that one thing I do not need is a problem. So I will be sitting on the edge of my chair to see what happens.

Today I planted impatiens in the backyard and calla lilies on the side. Swinging the maddox was quite a challenge. I had to stop to get my breath several times—low hemoglobin. But I did it!

It is now 6:15 p.m. and still light. This is my favorite time of the year. Everything is perched for blossoming. It is the season of hope for the future and what is sure to come. Perhaps I, too, am "perched!"

Virginia's long-term struggle with thrombocytopenia and anemia illustrates one of the challenges of a phase 1 trial. As a phase 1 patient you are always first to experience anything, and solutions take longer because your care providers have to figure out what is happening. If and when they do discover what is going on and what needs to be changed, they then have to get permission to alter the original protocol, which is typically written fairly conservatively. We already had the example of

Virginia's ANC and the protocol that required a suspension of drug at 1.5, which threshold was then changed to 1. Now Virginia's platelets began to drop. They dropped from a pre-STI 571 count of almost (800) 800,000 to less than (50) 50,000. You can survive and function at a platelet count of 35 if you are careful not to bruise, cut yourself or fall. However, the trial protocol mandated that if a patient dropped below 50, they had to go off the drug until they rebounded to 75. At a count below 50, Virginia would go off the drug. Three weeks later she would reach 75 and go back on. Eventually Dr. Sawyers was able to allow her to go down to 35 before she went off and only up to 50 before going back on. Even with the adjustments, Virginia would be on platelet-induced cycles for a year until her platelets settled into the low 50s. The March 17, 2000 biopsy registered 70 percent normal cells, and the 12/12 translocation was gone. The biopsy in July 2000 showed 85 percent normal cells with no evidence of the 12/12 translocation. The September biopsy was the same as July. The two of us proclaimed the 12/12 translocation gone forever, and it was.

But Virginia's troubles with anemia were returning. The drug Procrit would have stimulated red blood cell production, but in the early years the study doctors thought that there was a real possibility that a red blood cell stimulant might accelerate the production of leukemia cells, so they refused to change the protocol to allow its use. Subsequent studies showed that Procrit did no harm to CML patients who needed it; but Virginia didn't get it for a few years, and for the years she was refused it, she also cycled on and off the STI 571 in order to avoid transfusions. She was paying for all this cycling with bone marrow tests that showed that the situation had stabilized with CML still present.

The slowing progress toward "no detectable disease" caused us both to worry about what all this cycling was doing to the effectiveness of the treatment. Some researchers added to our worry by speculating that cycling on and off might encourage the development of resistant forms of CML.

April 2, 2000: I should have received my bone marrow results by now. I'm reticent to call UCLA. I'm afraid of what I'll find out.

April 4, 2000: Called UCLA—bone marrow results good—but I was hoping for better. 70 percent normal cells, 30 percent PH+. No other clones—the 12/12 thing is not there. What a relief.

Between April 14 and 21, we traveled to London and the South of France. In the context of what we had gone through, it was a sweet trip. We spent a lot of time with friends who had expected Virginia to die and now were able to partake of the miracle.

May 10, 2000: Well, there's yet another wrinkle in the fabric of life. My platelets are low—they plunged to 45 last Monday. Up to 51 Wednesday. Down to 48 this Monday.

They're now below 50 and UCLA has to take me off the drug. It's a big pain. I wonder, will the catch be that I won't be able to up my dosage to wipe out the last of the pesky PH+ cells? Ginny told me they were ready to put me on 400 mg when this platelet thing happened. It's a big pain in the rear. But I must think of it as only temporary.

I'm thankful for:

My little sweet little dog Bonnie Sue who's still hanging in.

My mother, who's doing really well.

Van, who continues to love me unconditionally even though my life causes him so much inconvenience and worry.

May 28, 2000: My blood stabilized the week before last. Platelets up to 56, white cells at 3.3. My reaction of relief was accompanied by a concern: "Are my white cells out of control?" It's really interesting, that reaction. There are so many things to worry about.

—What will my next BMB say?

—Will I ever get rid of the PH+ cells? If I do, will it stay that way?

—Will this cancer develop a resistance to STI 571? Or is it finally the answer?

—Will I live or will I die? Sometimes I feel like I'm walking on the edge of a profound abyss. I am anxious and pray the earth doesn't crumble under my feet and send me to my death.

In the beginning of this new experience, I was just grateful for a respite from interferon/ARA-C therapy; now I realize how devastated I will be if this drug fails. I continue, however, to feel in my gut that STI 571 is all it so far seems to be.

It is interesting to me that I function every day as if I'm not facing the terrible threat that looms before me. I never think about it most days—a survival mechanism?

I thank everyone for my feeling of well-being and normalcy. It is truly the greatest gift of all.

Like everyone else in my predicament, I'm sure I can't stop asking, why did this happen to me? I feel compelled to find out what I did to cause this, even though it's counterproductive.

Then, much to my surprise, Virginia called me while I was on the way back from a management retreat and told me that she had signed us up to run/walk the March 2001 Los Angeles Marathon as a fundraiser for The Leukemia & Lymphoma Society. I hung up and turned to my colleague Simon Berneau and told him what she had done. I told him that she had said, "You're not going to turn me down! I have leukemia." Within a day, Simon and his wife had made a generous contribution to our fundraising and signed up for the marathon on their own.

5.

Gleevec, Let the Marathons Begin

Through all her bouts with this terminal disease, Virginia and I went on with our lives. We went to work; we took care of our animals and each other. We saw friends. We traveled. Sure we were scaled back; it wasn't the life we had previously. But in all of this, Virginia served as a model for others. The students she taught felt they shared in her victory, and the other patients she met took inspiration from her. One day at work Virginia got a call from Virginia Ruvelcaba, a seventy-year-old from El Monte who had been watching CNN and saw Virginia and learned that she worked at Diamond Bar High School. She had CML too, and she tracked Virginia down so she could find out how she could get "that drug." This sweet, smart and aggressive lady captured a piece of our hearts. Every time she called she said, "Hello Virginia, this is the other Virginia." Mrs. Ruvelcaba was not a wealthy person and had no prescription insurance. As difficult as it was to find a way to get the drug for the "other Virginia," with Virginia's help she was ultimately able to get it through a program sponsored by Novartis.

We received a call from Dr. Sawyers asking if Virginia would mind accompanying him to a meeting of UCLA's Jonssen Cancer Center Board of Trustees. The meeting was designed, like most trustee meetings, to encourage them to give more money to the cancer program at the center. Virginia described the benefits of STI 571 and what it had done for the quality of her life.

June 1, 2000: We went to the Regency Club at the Penthouse at the corner of Westwood and Wilshire Boulevards so I could tell my story to the board of trustees of the Jonnson Cancer Center at UCLA. Dr. Sawyers gave a scientific presentation on STI 571 and was as excited as a kid in a candy store. I talked about my experience with STI 571. Several people come up and said how touched they were. I was nervous, but I guess I did OK. Van said I was awesome, but he's biased. Dustin Hoffman is a board member but he had the audacity not to come even though he knew I was to speak! Dr. Sawyers gave me a hug. I was deeply touched.

—One week until my next bone marrow biopsy. I know it will be a better report than last time.

—My platelets are down in the 40s again—no calls from UCLA—no symptoms.

—White count is 4.4 one time. That makes me nervous! Next time it's down in the 3's.

I'm thankful for:

My healthy and happy Bonnie.

My sweet Annie, who is slowly mellowing out.

My Van, whose shoulder is getting better.

My mother, who's enjoying life again.

Van's mother Sammy, who continues to improve after her operation.

Connie and the boys, who always entertain and support me.

June 23, 2000: UCLA called to say my BMB changed to nine thirty with Dr. Paquette. I called back and said no and demanded an appointment with Sawyers on June 28. Now I had two more days to wait.

I'm very uneasy, anticipating pain and results. May things be better.

Platelets still in the 40s but white count at 3.3. Hemoglobin is still down—8.1.

I feel these will bottom out soon and I'll be in good shape.

At the July biopsy, Dr. Sawyers said that after Virginia left the meeting, the trustees opened up their checkbooks. Dr. Sawyers, who we later found out had a lucrative offer elsewhere, could stay. We had him for some more time and we needed him desperately. With her biopsy wound bandaged up and the two of them ready to say goodbye, Virginia extended her hand, but instead Dr. Sawyers gave her a big hug. We had thought we had a partner in her treatment; now we knew.

July 22, 2000: On the day of my bone marrow test, they caught up with me and my low platelets. That day they were 46. They took me off the drug until they go up to 75. Today was the first day back on—three weeks to the day. It made me very unsettled to be off the drug, especially when I found out my bone marrow test results: 85 percent normal. Steady and constant improvement. Dr. Sawyers put me up to 400 mg, so maybe things will get even better. If persistence, will, and single-mindedness can do it, I'm in good shape.

It strikes me how odd, as well as poignant, it is that while I'm living this little intense life-and-death drama, the world goes about its business. Sometimes it makes me feel so small and insignificant, and I guess it demonstrates that in the larger picture, indeed I am. I always try to push myself out of that place quickly, though, because I know there's nothing good to gain from those thoughts.

P.S. Dr. Sawyers said after I left they pulled out their checkbooks at the trustees' meeting.

P.P.S Dr. Sawyers said goodbye and instead of taking my extended hand, he hugged me. I am blessed.

July 29, 2000: Van is in China now. Left yesterday and comes back next Wednesday. I miss him terribly. He is so important to my well-being in my daily life. May he be kept safe and return unharmed.

What will my blood test say Monday? Will my platelets have plunged after being on 400 mg for a week? Another person in the Internet discussion group achieved 100 percent normal cells—for two bone marrow tests! She went in for the next one and Dr. Sawyers said she didn't need it. She had a FISH (fluorescence in situ hybridization) test that showed 0 percent PH+ cells. Because the FISH test is even more sensitive than bone marrow, he said she was released to have blood tests once a month, but that she doesn't have to come back to UCLA. This was news that she said made her happy, yet uneasy. I can relate. Dr. Druker is back in the lab trying to figure out why some people achieve total cytogenetic response while others do not. May he find out soon.

August 20, 2000: My dear fur child Bonnie is in a bad place. She really doesn't want to eat—even my homemade custard that I make her for breakfast. She'd always eats that and now she doesn't want it. We made her roast beef, steak, chicken liver, chicken, etc., and she turns it all down. Who knows what's going on?

I'm thankful for:

My sweet Bonnie still hanging in there.

Still feeling good.

Being able to work out four times a week.

Van's support.

Mother still hanging in.

September 3, 2000: Well, I had a big shock a few moments ago. Van told me he is taking Professor Ding flying tomorrow. He'll be gone all day—on my birthday! I know I may be acting a bit childish, but I can't believe he did this. Here I was relishing the thought of spending a day with him. I'm so disappointed and hurt. But I suppose I'll get over it.

Van has been very withdrawn lately. He always held his feelings close, but these days it's worse. If I ask him what's wrong or what's going on, he refuses to acknowledge anything is wrong and becomes quite annoyed. I feel shut out.

I suppose spending my birthday alone is not the end of the world. I will simply have to adapt and overcome. I always do.

October 24 at 3:00 a.m.: Van's mother Sammy up and died. She told Don she felt kind of "flu-ish" off and on since the previous Thursday. Finally at 7 p.m., he took her to the emergency room with a fever of 100 something. She was admitted to the hospital and taken to ICU where she died at 3 a.m. Cause of death: unknown. But she was bleeding into her catheter bag all that time. Don didn't want an autopsy. The coroner didn't investigate. The death certificate, after three weeks of three doctors refusing to sign it, says atherosclerosis. She was seventy-nine. Her death has been devastating to all, including my mother. Don is barely making it. Connie and Van are back and forth trying to ease his pain and make him eat, which is hard for him to do.

My mother, after several months of serious depression and over-medicating herself, decided she needed to go to Knollwood Psychiatric and Chemical Dependency Center, which she did four weeks ago tomorrow. Sammy's death sent her over the edge. When I went out to

Hemet to take her to the hospital in Riverside, she didn't answer the door. I found her lying in a fetal position across her bed, barely able to talk. After two weeks there and a bit of recovery from drug haze, she announced she wasn't going back home. She wanted to go into an assisted living facility where she will be completely taken care of. So Van and I have spent many hours on finding such a place for her. She will be going to Valley Christian Home soon.

My bone marrow biopsy took four weeks to get results. I knew something was strange when we actually got the cytogenetic report. It said 70 percent normal cells. But there had also been a FISH test done. It said 82 percent normal cells. This was quite a blow. After expecting maybe 100 percent normal I get this? Questioning begins. Why? Am I slipping? — Is something really bad beginning to happen? The wondering, the worrying. We decided an 82 percent FISH test is good and more accurate than a 20-cell biopsy. I sit on the edge of my seat waiting for December 18 when I have my next one.

I decided that I needed to go to the December 2000 American Association of Hematology annual meeting in San Francisco. We had the right drug, but why was it driving platelets and hemoglobin counts down? Were there others with the same problems? Were there other treatments in the works in case this one went wrong? I was deep into the literature and couldn't find answers. Maybe I could learn more from freshly presented articles or from the anecdotal side of the presentations.

From my point of view, the ASH annual meeting of the year 2000 was a watershed. I was frankly amazed by how much research had been done in the year and a half since the trial had begun. It was becoming obvious that researchers were realizing that there were quiescent cells in the marrow that were left untouched by STI571 because the drug only dealt with cells that differentiated and proliferated, and the quiescent cells did not. Papers suggested that growth factors such as (GM-CSF) could be used to cause differentiation in combination with STI571 that would control the proliferation. One presenter suggested that off-and-on-again application of STI 571 might bring out the quiescent cells.

For the first time, I heard about the PCR test, which was much more sensitive than bone marrow tests. The PCR tests would prove to be our obsession for the next seven years.

It was clear to researchers that STI 571 was not proving effective against advanced disease. And it was also clear that some people were resisting. My most vivid memory of the conference came when Dr. Sawyers, standing in front of a 30-foot projection of himself, said to an audience of more than 1,000 people that what they had to do now was figure out what to do when patients experience resistance to STI 571. He added that this was essential because experience shows that resistance will come. He had never told us this when we were in his office. The reality of Dr. Sawyers' statement frightened me, but his team had already found the answer. They already knew that mutations were causing the pockets in the protein that held STI 571 to change shape, preventing STI 571 from bonding and letting ATP back in.

Those who spoke recommended that patients never go off the drug unless they had to. We had to find a way to stabilize Virginia's anemia so she could stay on the drug all the time. There was a fascinating presentation on a combination SRC, ABL inhibitor that better fit into the BCR-ABL protein's pocket. Still, at this conference, the buzz was STI 571. There were papers or presentations on twenty-four other suggested treatments for CML; and although the SRC, ABL inhibitor foretold the future, it was clear to me that STI 571 administered at UCLA by Dr. Sawyers was our ticket to health and happiness. Not only did the team there understand the nuances of how this drug worked, but they were anticipating problems and finding solutions for them. I didn't know that Dr. Sawyers was already lining up a study for a SRC, ABL inhibitor that showed tremendous promise.

I also learned how remarkable it was that Novartis had gone ahead with the drug's development. Other companies also had inhibitors in the pipeline. Pfizer was allowing researchers to test a SRC inhibitor that showed great promise, as eloquently explained in a poster paper written by researchers from Moffitt Cancer Center in Florida. When I talked to the authors, however, it was clear that Pfizer was not likely to go beyond this small study. Where was the money to be made? Obviously frustrated, the researchers suggested I write a letter to the company. The conference introduced me again to the confluence and conflict of the tenuous balance between profit motive and serving patients.

The meeting also gave me absolute confirmation that 400 mg of STI 571 was now considered the minimum standard dose. After my return and after Virginia's platelet counts were high enough to allow her back on the drug, we made sure it remained at 400 mg.

Almost as important as the confirmation that we had made the right treatment decision was my education about the celebrity doctors in CML research. You simply do not present at ASH unless your peers judge that you have something important to say. Melo, Sawyers, Talpaz, Holyoake, Druker, Gorre, Kantarjian—these names would be the center of my research for the future. When I could, I returned to the ASH annual meeting and I was never disappointed. The scientific facts I learned would lay the groundwork for my understanding of problems that I would be facing in the very near future.

January 7, 2001: I forgot one really big thing. In September I signed Van and myself up to walk the L.A. Marathon on March 4 for the Leukemia Society. We are responsible for raising $1,300 each in donations—so far we've raised $4,400 together. We train with a group of people from the San Gabriel Valley and our coach, Tina Escobar, every Sunday. We are up to fifteen miles, which takes us four hours and fifteen minutes. A different part of my body hurts each time we train. I have blisters on every part of my feet. We went to a running store so we have the right shoes and socks and shirts. We have "body glide" to prevent chafing—and boy do you need it!

When we hit ten miles, we began to "crap out" for the rest of the day. It's really a lost day. But we met some really nice people. Our coach runs 26.2 miles in less than three hours! Wow! She's forty-six and has run forty marathons. She's also very sweet and nonjudgmental. My hemoglobin is very low so the hills are very hard for me, but I do it! Dr. Sawyers says it's OK. Doing this training is a lot like getting through treatment with interferon. You just have to put one foot in front of the other and do the best you can.

Today a weird thing happened when I was walking by myself because Van's in Vietnam. I was on my way back to Bonelli Park on Puddingstone Drive when a car (old beige Nissan or something) with four men in it drove by. I had a weird intuition. They slowed down going by and I was all alone—no one else in sight—no houses either, just before the dam road turnoff. I prepared my plan for if they came back. They came back. I walked down the side of the road to another road leading to a parking lot—they followed on that road. I got my cell phone out, dialed 911 so I could hit send if I needed to and waited. I turned on the dam road—no car. But then a truck kept driving by, so paranoid as I was, I put my phone up to my ear every time a vehicle passed by. By the time I walked down the hill to meet the group in the park, the car came by again. When I told everyone about my experience, Tina and two guys took off to find the car. They didn't but reported it to the police. Wow!

I was kind of afraid to walk by myself and was just feeling confident when this happened. Oh well. It all turned out OK.

Signing up for a marathon put Virginia over the top as a model for others, including me. But oh man was that training hard for a fat old college administrator. Three, five, eight, ten, twelve, fifteen, eighteen, and twenty miles. Uphill, downhill, on paths and streets. Cold weather, hot weather, and rain. Blisters with old shoes. Blisters with the new ones. Barely able to get into the car to go home. Harder to get out. During all of this Virginia put her head down and pushed on, anemia and all. The example of Virginia's strength and the comparison with her fight against cancer was not lost on me or anyone on the team.

March 2, 2001 saw us lined up for the Los Angeles Marathon. We had trained almost every Saturday since September. Virginia had a hemoglobin level of 8.3, almost four points below normal, but she was ready. Still, it is impossible to describe the feeling when you go out on a course with 25,000 other people. We did what they call intervals. We would run one minute and then walk four. It is faster than walking, but not by a whole lot. Anyway the goal was to finish. Aside from the exhaustion part, marathons are a hoot. During this one, Virginia first found our great teammate and friend Jacquie Ochoa Rossellini. Jacquie, a beautiful young woman, an accountant, had trained with us and by her own testimonial took great inspiration from Virginia. She walked with us for the whole marathon. The experience was made more interesting by the fact that Virginia was chosen to be a featured participant and was interviewed on the course. Her feature was then shown live on television. She showed her enthusiasm for being alive and able to walk the L.A. marathon for others. Jacquie and I slipped in and out of the picture.

After the interview, thirteen miles into the course, we found one of our teammates sitting on a curb. Frank was walking for his young son who had leukemia. He was a truck driver whose schedule kept him from a lot of training, and his shoes were way past their prime. He was exhausted and had blisters the size of silver dollars. Virginia walked over to him and said, "Frank, you have to get up and walk in with us. You have to do this for your son." And that is exactly what he did. We all walked across the finish line holding hands—a pretty motley crew—but Frank's family was so proud of him. He was forever grateful to Virginia. Jacquie already loved Virginia; this just put another dimension to that love. I know how she feels.

April 12, 2001: I'm on the airplane heading for Shanghai, China. I took two personal days and will be gone all next week (my spring break.)

Highlights of the past three months:

—Sue Dilks presenting us with a care package for marathon.

—Twenty-mile walks that killed my feet.

—Staying at the Biltmore Hotel the night before the marathon.

—Speaking at the pasta dinner after Mayor Riordan and making my teammates cry when I spoke of Van feeding me through a straw.

—Sue Dilks, nurse at the cancer center and fellow Team in Training member, showing up at the Biltmore before the L.A. Marathon and taking photos of all of us.

—Walking the marathon for eight hours and twenty-two minutes—my knee beginning to hurt a lot at about mile 15—keeping Frank going even though he had blisters all over his feet—being interviewed by UPN 13—the official live coverage of the marathon—two

weeks before and at the marathon with my little Honored Hero, Corey, the cutest little boy who was fighting acute lymphocytic leukemia.

—Corey coming up to me at the pasta dinner and hugging me—a big bear hug.

—Jacquie Ochoa-Rossellini sticking with us the whole way.

—Getting to mile 20 and saying to myself "only 6.2 miles left"—the longest 6.2 miles I've ever walked.

—Being chased onto the sidewalk by police and the street sweepers and not wanting to walk up and down the driveways.

—Wondering where the 26-mile marker was for it seemed like 10 miles. (It never came).

—Limping with my left knee and my right foot with a dollar-sized blister.

—Going around the last corner to see the finish line and bursting into tears of relief and joy.

—Joining hands with Van, Jacquie and Frank, and seeing nephew Stephen filming us with my tears of joy and exhilaration.

—The lady putting the medal around my neck.

—The other lady taking off my electronic timing chip.

—Walking the .2 mile back to the Biltmore and crying again when Stephen showed me the UPN 13 video and his finish-line video.

—Taking a nice soak in the bathtub in the hotel room.

—Coming home to various phone messages of congratulations from people who saw me on TV.

—Going to work March 5 and basking in my glory all day.

—Meeting Van at the Cancer Center for my weekly blood test and basking in my glory there with Sue Dilks presenting me with a photo album of all the pictures she took.

—Driving to a Mexican restaurant to celebrate with a beer and dinner. Stopping at the light by Albertsons with Van stopped behind me. Van was slammed into by a van going 40 mph with no brakes—Van's car stopped her—his car hit me and then slammed into the car stopped next to us in the other lane.

—I remember Van's airbag going off and bruising and burning his

arm and him going back to the van and saying to the driver, "You rear-ended me" and her responding, "I did not!"

—Calling Frank and Connie, Frank and Stephen coming to get us, the police and tow truck driver saying, "Oh, oh, oh, those two cars are totaled."

—Being very angry that my "day" had been rained on and fighting that negativity.

I think this first marathon let the doctors see Virginia differently. She obviously functioned on low hemoglobin. We didn't let anyone know how hard that was for her, but she now was allowed to stay on the drug.

Other STI 571 trials were initiated and advanced until Novartis had enough positive information to prove to the FDA that the drug worked. There was an awkward period between the end of trials and the drug's approval by the FDA. Trial centers, which had now grown to dozens, were scurrying to get their documents in order with their t's crossed and i's dotted. Those who had participated in the trials would still get the drug but it was unavailable to anyone else who needed it. It actually was a desperate time for some, but on May 10, 2001, the FDA approved STI 571 for the treatment of CML. It had been the fastest approval process in the history of the FDA. STI 571 became the drug Gleevec.

May 20, 2001: On the leukemia front, STI 571 was approved for general use on Thursday, May 10, 2001. This news was really big and CNN did yet another story on me. They even called me at school and did a live interview. It's kind of a kick in the pants. The drug is now on pharmacists' shelves and will cost $2,300 to $2,800 depending on the dose. Wow! I feel proud to have had a part in this and happy to be on the road to being "better." My next bone marrow test is June 4 and being normal, I am anxious about the results. Also anxious about what will happen to my relationship with Dr. Sawyers now that it's been approved. Time will tell.

The FDA approved STI 571 not only for the treatment of CML but also for the treatment of a terminal disease, Gastrointestinal Stromal Tumors (GIST), for which it was not designed. It turned out that STI

571 also inhibited another protein called C-KIT whose cancerous version was the culprit in GIST. The wife of a very wealthy man from Finland had GIST, and he came to believe that he might be able to save her with STI 571. With his considerable resources, he obtained a supply of STI 571 and funded a Dana Farber clinical trial for his wife. The results were as remarkable for GIST as they were for CML. I like to think of this as a love story. It also saved thousands of people who suffered from a cancer that otherwise would have resulted in the surgical removal of their stomach parts and then inevitable death.

After the approval of Gleevec, all but the phase 1 trial CML patients were cut loose to buy their own supply of the drug. Virginia and her phase 1 colleagues were technically still on the trial as researchers tracked their progress; they would be given drugs for the remainder of their lives. Lucky as they were, and albeit motivated first by their own survival, Virginia and all those who participated in the phase 1 trial were pioneers for many people. Ed Crandall had already lost his life. My friend Peter Rowbotham, despite his brilliant fight against it, would eventually lose his wife, Rita. David Lawyer would die as well. These people's legacy was a better understanding of a drug that gave hope and life to thousands of people.

I was just hooked on marathons and next I hooked my sixteen-year-old nephew, Stephen, and Virginia's sixty-three year-old cousin Tom into training for and doing the Rock 'n' Roll Marathon in June in San Diego. Both these guys had stuck with us during the worst of times. Besides having breakfast with us once a week and videoing us during the Los Angeles Marathon, Stephen was deeply fascinated by the science of Virginia's disease and even filmed one of Virginia's bone marrow tests for a science project. Tom is as close to a brother as Virginia will ever have.

At San Diego, Stephen and I lost track of Tom. Within the context of 25,000 people, this turns out to be pretty easy to do, especially if someone takes an unannounced potty break. Stephen and I decided to pace ourselves by following a very old gentleman we were sure we could pass when the time came. We should have known that we had miscalculated when we read "Las Vegas Running Club" on the old guy's T-shirt. As the fellow pulled away from us, he left us exhausted and wondering how we were going to get to the finish line. I had to stop Stephen from taking off his shoes at mile 17 then from sitting one inch past the line when we finally finished. He got himself to the medical tent where they fixed him up with liquids and food. Even then, he was a mess and decided to sit down about ten yards after leaving the medical tent. When I reached down to pull him up off the tarmac, he assured me that if I tried, he would throw up on me. Still, while it took me three days to recover, Stephen was fine an hour later. Damned kids. Stephen and I had a very respectable time for walkers, and it proved to be my lifetime personal best. For his part, Tom came in a few minutes later with his lifetime personal best. From this time on, Tom, Virginia, and I became a walking team. Stephen had more common sense and retired. I realized from a recent conversation that he still brags about his time. Sweet boy to do a marathon with me. I remain proud of him for the feat.

Though the marathons kept us in good spirits, and Virginia appeared to be winning her battle with CML, the level of anxiety was not over for us—would Gleevec work over time? Would Virginia eventually relapse? What were the mechanisms for relapse? Would BCR-ABL find new communication pathways? Would the protein mutate? We had moments of joy, but very few moments of peace. I spent my time learning computer animation programs and animating the entire process that made STI 571 work. I even began to develop an animation of how resistance worked through mutation of BCR-ABL.

As if to put a period to the joyful days of beating back CML, our dog Bonnie died in Bridgeport on August 10. I loved this dog, but she was Virginia's canine soul mate.

August 11, 2001: How could this be? How can she be forever gone? I still can't grasp it. My pain continues. My heart is in pieces, my panic often, my feelings of loss so deep, right now I don't feel I'll ever mend.

I see that sweet little face with those kind eyes before me, and I melt into tears. I look for her taking a nap. I see the emptiness of the kitchen floor with no beds and no food "shelf" to help her eat. I yearn to pet her soft body and to cradle her little face in my hands and place it next to mine—to kiss her little forehead and nose. But I can never do that again. I am devastated.

September 8, 2001: Dear Bonnie Sue,

Even though you have gone, I feel your presence every day. Today in the grocery, I noted how strange it is to not worry about buying milk and eggs for your custard, Boost for your ice cream, or meat and baby food. My heart broke all over again as I realized these things were no longer needed.

Bonnie, I miss you so desperately. I miss your patient personality, your cuddling, your hugs, your sweet personality, your big brown kind eyes, your flowing hair.

The new schnauzer, Rosie, isn't like you. She bites all the time; she's bitten through the phone cord twice and chewed through the cell-phone battery charger cords too—she doesn't like to cuddle—she sleeps at the front of the bed. I miss your sweet little body cuddled up next to mine. And Bonnie, I knew all the time I had you that I probably would never have that again. In a way, that's good. It makes you very unique. I knew that too.

You are my sweetheart. I will always love you. You are a part of me forever. You are always with me.

Your mama,
Ginny

6.

I Can't Believe This is Happening: Metastatic Melanoma

Bonnie's death not only reminded us that life is fragile and that Virginia's situation had to be put in that context, but it also served as a mental cue for the beginning of events that would again turn our lives upside down.

Right around the time of Bonnie's loss, I felt a strange bump the size of a BB on the top of my head. Initially, I thought it was a pimple, but it didn't go away. Eventually, I trundled down to the dermatologist to have it looked at. He seemed unconcerned, but did take it out to have it biopsied. At that point, he let me know that it might have more significance than he first thought. Two and a half weeks later, over the phone, at work, I was told that little bump was melanoma. I had always thought melanomas were on the surface of the skin, so I didn't understand how mine could have been under it. Well, melanoma does indeed start cutaneously, or on the top of the skin. But when it starts to spread, it can go anywhere; and when it does, the cancer term is that it has metastasized, and metastatic melanoma is a disease that kills most people within a few years.

The dermatologist said they could not help me and that I needed to go to either Norris Cancer Center at USC where I would find Dr. Jeffrey Weber or to John Wayne Cancer Institute at Saint John's Health Center where I would find Dr. Donald Morton. Not only would I find the best doctors at these two institutions, but I would also find the clinical trials I needed. By now, I didn't have to do research to understand the implications of these instructions.

I told my friend and colleague Daryl about the call I had just received and that I was going to see Virginia who was having a blood test at the cancer center. He drove me to her. When I arrived, Virginia could read my face and then the quiver in my voice as I told her that I had metastatic melanoma. Understandably, she freaked and told anyone who would listen that if I died, she would stop taking her medicine and die too; there was nothing anyone could do to stop her. The oncology psychologist was front and center in a flash. This was not going the way I expected. I was in big trouble. We were both in big trouble.

October 22, 2001: I'm sitting at the Robert and Beverly Lewis Cancer Care Center having my blood test, talking to Nancy and Vicki when I look up and there in the doorway stands Van—like he's done so many times before. With beer and Mexican food on my mind I say, "Oh, there's my Prince Charming!" Then I notice Darryl standing next to Van, and I notice the strained look on his face. I jump up, run over, and ask what's wrong. Van tells me the lump taken off his head two and a half weeks before came back as metastatic melanoma.

My midsection was slashed by blue lightning and I felt my face drain of blood. My legs got rubbery and Nancy the nurse ran over and sat me down. My mind was a flurry of questions—isn't my leukemia enough? How will I go on if Van dies? This isn't fair! How did this happen?

Dr. Weber, the first doctor recommended by dermatologist, was doing interesting work developing advanced techniques to stimulate immune responses to melanoma. He was well published and managed a team of people with an impressive array of skills. He also had quite a reputation administering what was then a relatively new treatment for melanoma called biochemotherapy in which the biological agents interferon and Interleukin-2 are added to a line of chemotherapy agents to make an infusion cocktail so challenging to the human body that it had to be administered in the hospital. Dr. Weber's program was also part of the USC Norris Cancer Center, a comprehensive cancer center. This meant that a group of people, with different talents, worked together at one place treating cancer patients. We would later come to understand how useful this would be.

Dr. Morton at John Wayne Cancer Institute was legendary for his work on cancer. He had invented the sentinel node biopsy. This procedure begins with a radioactive dye being injected into a tumor site. The spreading dye is tracked until it hits the first lymph node. That lymph node is removed and biopsied to see if it contains cancer cells. If it does, more lymph nodes are removed from a sequence of lymph nodes until the surgeon finds a clear one. Done right, the surgery stops with the one or two clear lymph nodes, and the surgeon sews things up avoiding the removal of unnecessary ones. But the original melanoma is removed. This procedure is used extensively for patients with breast cancer as well as melanoma and has saved a lot of people unnecessary surgery and disfigurement.

At the time I had to make my decision, Dr. Morton was also very well known for his proprietary experimental melanoma vaccine, Canvaxin, that he claimed had extended the lives of many, many people. This polyvalent vaccine was made from a number of cancer tumors, processed together to create a drug introduced through an infusion. The assertion was that out of all the tumors processed, one will activate the patient's immune system against their specific tumor. Canvaxin had not been approved by the FDA, but Dr. Morton was quite convincing in his promotion of both the vaccine and his company that manufactured it.

One of the nurses who had helped Virginia for many years told us that her brother had been diagnosed with melanoma and had gone to John Wayne and with treatment there, had survived for eighteen years.

I ultimately chose John Wayne because it too administered biochemotherapy. The doctor in charge of this program was Dr. Steven O'Day, a person nearly as respected as Dr. Weber.

I made my appointment with Dr. Morton. Virginia and I always got along with Dr. Morton, but given his prominence, we found ourselves entirely on his terms. We were put in an exam room at 9:15 a.m. and he showed up at 1:45 p.m. When it came to the surgery, he insisted that before he would operate, we write him a personal check for $4,000 even though we had excellent insurance. We paid, and he operated.

I had the remains of a bump on my head and needed to have it removed along with anything else the sentinel node biopsy pointed to. On October 25, 2001, I had a CT scan, an MRI, and a PET scan. Computerized tomography (CT) scans use X-rays, but instead of the two-dimensional image delivered by stationary X-rays, this one is three-dimensional. This is made possible by rotating the X-ray source around a tube in which the patient is situated. With the help of a computer, the result is a series of cross-sectional images of internal body structures including both organs and tumors. The patient usually drinks a radioactive material and over time, I witnessed a number of people throw it back up. Most often, another radioactive material is injected during the scan to increase contrast.

Magnetic resonance imaging (MRI) is used to see higher contrast between different soft tissues, and in my case it would be used to get a better image of the brain than we could get with a CT scan. Unlike the CT that uses radiation, the MRI uses a magnetic field to create the image. Nonradioactive contrast is often injected during the scan.

Positron emission tomography (PET) scans also give a three-dimensional look at the body. PET scans work on the principle that when the body is still, tumors are the predominant users of sugar. The process begins with a nurse injecting radioactive sugar into a patient who then lies down for an hour without moving. In theory, if the patient is then scanned for radiation hot spots, only the tumors will show up. To make the scan more accurate, they often combine it with a CT scan. I never liked these scans much, and there are ways to mess them up. I learned the hard way that you should not exercise before a scan because the little muscle tears will show up looking like tumors.

November 12, 2001: For the past three weeks, I have lived in hell. Van has had:

—CT scan of neck, abdomen, chest, pelvis.

—MRI of brain.

—PET scan full body.

—Ultrasound of liver.

—Eye exam (they pressed on his eyeballs).

—Chest X-ray.

Having ascertained the best doctor to go to, Donald Morton at John

*Wayne Cancer Institute at Saint John's Health Center, we traveled up
and down the Santa Monica Freeway to John Wayne Cancer Institute
(two hours each way for four different days.) I took three days off and
four afternoons off with people covering my sixth-period class.*

*We had an appointment Thursday November 1 to hear the results of
the tests. That day it took two and a half hours to get in for a nine fifteen
appointment. We were taken to an exam room and waited there until 1:45
p.m. I thought I would die, but this time from grief and overload rather
than cancer. When the doctor came in at one forty-five, he told us the
results were all negative, so they would treat the spot on Van's head as
a primary site. They would do a wide excision of the area, put on a skin
graft from his thigh, do a sentinel node test where they take out the lymph
node the radioactive dye drains to and check for cancer, and take off a
small lump on his right arm.*

*It was a relief. But where these melanoma cells came from was
a mystery. The lump on his head was the size of a bb and under the
skin—no mole. That's why this whole thing is such a shock.*

*I can't believe this is happening. It seems to me that the cross Van
and I have had to bear for four years should be enough. But no, here's
yet another challenge of the highest order for you to deal with. I know we
can do it—we have a proven track record—but there comes a time when
you just feel weary. CANCER SUCKS.*

On November 12, starting at 7 a.m., I got the radioactive dye to
see which lymph node it would go to. It took longer than expected, but
finally the dye reached its target and I was off for surgery. Dr. Morton
removed three lymph nodes in my neck and a suspicious lump on my
arm and had them biopsied. I would later find out that all four were
negative. He next removed the melanoma on my head and a four-inch
circle of flesh around it. He sent these out for biopsy. More good news:
The center was positive, but the surrounding tissue was not. He then took
a patch of skin from my thigh, processed it, and then sewed it on top
of my head where my hair had been. I instantly became a partially bald
old guy. I woke up with a big wound on my thigh and a wad of treated
gauze called a bolster stapled to my head. Over the bolster were layers

of Vaseline-soaked sheets of gauze and then a mesh cap to hold it all in place. There was so much height to all this that I looked like a cone head. We went home at 10:00 p.m. I was hoping that this was all worth it and wondering how I was going to sleep without ripping the bandages apart. The only thing that hurt was my thigh. I was so exhausted that I didn't think much about what Virginia had been through.

November 12, 2001: Veterans Day. Connie drove us in to St. John's Hospital to be there for Van's surgery. Since it is a holiday, we left at 6 a.m. and got there at 7 a.m., one and a half hours early. No traffic.

8:30 a.m. Register.

9:15 a.m. Lymph node blue dye imaging in nuclear medicine.

11:00 a.m. Back to room in presurgery area.

1:15 p.m. Taken to surgery.

We're waiting. Questions flying into each other in my head—will he die on the table? Will the lymph node be clear? Will the lump on his arm be melanoma? Will the pain be excruciating?

3:45 p.m. Dr. Morton comes to find me. The lump on his arm is just fatty stuff. Three nodes were taken out.

Pathologist he really trusts said it could be a primary tumor scratched off.

Thursday we'll know results of nodes.

Still have lots to worry about.

By this time Gleevec had driven Virginia's hemoglobin down to 8.7, so she was really beat when she drove me home. In bed, I carefully positioned my head on the pillow, looked over, and saw Virginia was already dead to the world. The next day, despite the exhausting events, Virginia had to get up and go to work. I stayed home wondering what would happen if the graft didn't take. Two days later, we went back to Santa Monica to get my wounds checked by a nurse who also taught us how to change the bandages. She claimed that she knew a patient who had learned how to do this alone using mirrors. To this day, I don't see how that could have been possible. Luckily, I had Virginia who was hardening herself to deal with my head, which was at this time quite gruesome. Working together we rebandaged me at the hospital and were fairly confident that we could do it on our own the next day and every day thereafter. Mr. Cone Head and his beautiful anemic leukemia survivor wife found their way to the car and prepared to find the supplies we would need to rebandage me in the future. Anemia had put Virginia back into the oops period of driving. She had several fender benders as she would sometimes lose her ability to concentrate. On the way home from John Wayne, I had trouble adjusting the mass of bandages; she turned to help me as we drove down the Santa Monica freeway. As she did so, she drove up the rear end of a Toyota pickup. When we took down the driver's information, he never took his eyes off of me. That, by the way, was still not the most expensive of these accidents. That happened when she backed the car out of the carport with the back door open. The back door caught the main support for the carport and ripped it out. I still wonder why the carport roof held up.

After a few days, I went back to work at Cal Poly Pomona. We were building a new 10 million dollar building, and that and the general business of a university atmosphere required my presence. So cone head and all, I found myself back at work.

On December 6, I returned to John Wayne and had the bolster unstapled and was told that we could stop rebandaging my head. On that day, I was off to my second ASH annual meeting, this time in Orlando. My wound was still pretty hideous, but friends and coworkers kindly gave me a large collection of hats. I settled on a brown felt Australian hat, packed my bags, and headed for Florida.

December 6, 2001: All tests came back negative for Van. Nodes clear, tissue clear about the lump, etc. I have had to change his head gauze and bandage every morning—getting up earlier! Yea. So far so good.

Today at his second follow-up appointment, he was told he didn't have to wear the bandage anymore and they took out the staples. That's very good because he was off to the ASH conference in Orlando to find out about the latest leukemia stuff for me. He was worried about changing the bandages himself—but now he doesn't have to do it!

The 2001 ASH meeting was abuzz with papers and presentations on CML. I was worried about Virginia's low platelets, her anemia, and the possible consequences of her going on and off the drug. I finally met Peter Rowbotham in person. He was still trying to find solutions for Rita, whose challenges were multiplying. Dr. Sawyers was part of numerous presentations, and he was able to bring and showcase some of his research team. Also from UCLA, Dr. Neil Shah presented on the problem of relapse that was occurring in a subset of patients. Dr. Shah would one day become a friend and a star in his own right. Using new information from a paper by Dr. John Kuriyan of UC Berkeley about how STI 571 bound to BCR-ABL protein, Dr. Shah talked about the protein's ability to mutate its crystalline structure and thus block Gleevec's ability to bind into its intended pocket. The number of mutations so far discovered was in the dozens, but more were showing up as the number of Gleevec-treated patients increased. The lab was finding a solution for the mutations, except for one, called T315I, which was especially resistant to drugs. Dr. Shah would play a pivotal role in finding a drug to get this killer as well.

It became clear that the development and introduction of Gleevec had opened a floodgate of interest and research. There were 504 abstracts dealing with CML and 319 with Gleevec. The ASH conference had never seen anything as electrifying. Unfortunately, it has not seen anything like it since.

I was, however, uneasy. There was almost no discussion about some of the problems we had faced. No one wants to be a unique person in a cohort. There was no talk about anemia or low platelets as side effects, or what happens when treatment forces a person to go off the drug. There were papers that confirmed that in almost all cases residual disease remained, even with successful Gleevec treatment, and that in people removed from the drug, eventually the disease had come back. There were also articles about Gleevec failures. It did not work for Acute Lymphocytic Leukemia or BCR-ABL positive Acute Myelogenous Leukemia, and it didn't work for most CML patients beginning Gleevec in advanced stages of the disease.

Walking through the exhibitor section of the hematology

conference with all the pharmaceutical paraphernalia, I had a revelation that would change my life. I was walking past the Chiron booth with my brown hat on when I saw a reference to melanoma. I don't know why Chiron had a melanoma display at a hematology conference. When I stopped, a very nice young woman asked me if I was interested in melanoma and I explained that I was and why. She asked me what my stage was. At this time, I didn't really know and uttered something that I now know didn't make much sense. In an act of pity and compassion, she gave me a CD on melanoma that featured Dr. Steven O'Day. I thanked her then, but I wish I could let her know that this one improbable act helped me immensely.

I needed to gather up my brown hat and get back to my treatment and work. I was worn down to the nub.

Back home, we allayed our fears by talking directly to Dr. Sawyers about the course of Virginia's treatment. He was by now not just Virginia's physician, but also her friend. He gave us comforting and detailed explanations about why Virginia's progress was going well, if not as fast as we wanted. At this time, we should have asked ourselves what Dr. Sawyers' fame in this field meant. It portended a future crisis for us.

December 17, 2001: My latest test—a peripheral FISH test—came back only 2.7 percent PH+! Yea.

Dr. Sawyers raised my dose to 600 mg. Hope next time things are even better.

I began to question whether I wanted to continue with Dr. Morton and John Wayne Cancer Institute. After my recovery, the staff began to talk to me about going into Dr. Morton's Canvaxin trial. By this time, I had done extensive research on this drug and learned that it had been around for a long time and it had not yet received FDA approval. There was a lot of hubbub about Canvaxin's imminent approval, but, as I read more and more, it became hard for me to believe that was really going to happen. Many melanoma specialists agreed and the level of criticism leveled at Canvanxin was increasing. I was looking at a heavily criticized drug. Plus, the trial being offered to me was a double-blind one in which half the patients were to receive a placebo.

Dr. Morton met with me and Virginia and told us about the successes of Canvaxin, but he also told me that because he had a financial interest in the drug, he could not manage the trial. He would turn me over to his team. We thanked him for the surgery and we never saw him again.

I became more uncomfortable when one of the trial team changed my staging so I would qualify for the trial. He may have thought he was doing me a favor, but my response was to call John Wayne Cancer Institute and let them know that I was going to pursue options other than Canvaxin. Amazingly, the staff had presumed that I would accept a spot on the trial and had already randomized me, meaning that they had already decided whether or not I was going to receive the drug. A very kind nurse let me know that if I had gone ahead with the Canvaxin trial, I would have received the placebo.

With stronger trial controls, it became obvious that the drug was of no benefit to participants and thus the Canvaxin trial eventually ended in failure. I dwell on the demise of this drug's development because it illustrates how important informed health care decisions can be. I walk around with the results of Dr. Morton's truly fine surgical skills, but if I had stuck with him through Canvaxin's failure, I could very well be dead now.

I was back on my own. At first, I began to look for a signal transduction inhibitor like the one we found for Virginia. In fact, I read with great interest a study in which Gleevec itself was given to melanoma patients. Some melanoma patients had elevated levels of the C-kit protein, and Gleevec inhibited C-kit as well as BCR-ABL.

Even though Gleevec did indeed inhibit C-kit in melanoma patients, the anecdotal evidence from the discussion lists indicated that rather than suppressing the disease, it might be setting it loose. Still, I had to make decisions and move forward. I decided that all that was left for me was biochemotherapy or a more advanced vaccine.

I had already watched the Chiron disc featuring Dr. O'Day of John

Wayne. In it, he spent a lot of time talking about biochemotherapy as a melanoma treatment. Basically this treatment assumes that the combination of biological agents and chemotherapy given in successive and repeated treatments could destroy the melanoma.

In the literature, there were two main players in biochemotherapy. One was Dr. O'Day and the other was Dr. Weber at USC/Norris Cancer Center. Although both these doctors are terrific, I was inclined to call Dr. Weber because not only was he practiced in the delivery of biochemotherapy, he was also well known for his research in targeted peptide vaccines that represented a very different approach from Dr. Morton's shotgun polyvalent vaccine. He also had dozens of clinical trials under his belt, so he might offer me options that I could not foresee.

Dr. Blayney was still Virginia's general oncologist. He double-checked Virginia's counts and progress, but he mainly served as a bright and informed consultant. I asked if I could be his patient as well, and he agreed. I began to get excellent advice that helped me find a new direction. It became clear that Dr. Blayney held Dr. Weber in the highest regard.

By January 2002, I had my first appointment with Dr. Weber and his staff. They lined me up for a series of blood tests, a CT scan, an MRI, and another PET scan. It seems that no one trusts the information that comes from someone else's hospital. You just have to take the tests all over again. The results of the tests were all negative, so I was technically free of melanoma because Dr. Morton had removed the one identifiable tumor. In fact, I had no evidence of disease (NED)—a more accurate term that recognizes that the cancer is probably still there but impossible to measure with current technology. Dr. Weber and I would have discussed one of his peptide vaccine trials, but because those trials need to accrue large numbers of people, they are designed for people with the most common HLA type 2; and I was not one of them. To be sure, Dr. Weber called a friend at the National Cancer Institute to see if anyone in the country was offering a trial for non-HLA 2 patients. Nope. But that may have been lucky. As of today, none of those vaccines does anything close to what Gleevec did for Virginia. They do benefit some of the patients, but as Dr. Weber would later say, vaccine research is a one-inch-at-a-time business. The breakthroughs can be small and can be the foundation for the next small breakthroughs. In a situation like this, it is best to be at the end of the line, not the beginning. We would have this message repeated by Dr. Sawyers in other circumstances.

Because I was NED at this point, starting biochemotherapy was called adjuvant therapy, meaning preventative therapy that attacks what we believe to still be there. Dr. Weber and I had a long discussion about whether I wanted to undergo this or wait until new melanoma popped up. I wanted to go ahead with the biochemotherapy right away. If this was to be our choice, then we needed to get on with it.

Virginia and I continued to work out together, but her hemoglobin was dropping, and it was getting very hard for her to continue. We had recently requested and been allowed to increase her dose from 400 mg to 600 mg. Although her leukemia load dropped dramatically as a result, by early January her hemoglobin had dropped to 7.8, a full two points below the point when most people got a transfusion. Seeing success, Virginia wanted to stay on the drug, and luckily for us Dr. Sawyers agreed to allow her to take the red blood cell stimulant Procrit in the hope that her hemoglobin counts would rise. It was clear by this time that blood stimulants would not stimulate the leukemia. It took three weeks before the counts began to rise. We felt hope for an end of this for Virginia.

In the meantime, Dr. Weber had referred me to one of his patients who was on a break between biochemotherapy treatments. He let me know that the treatment required that the patient be given a PICC line that went from the inside of the arm to the heart. It would stay in over the course of all the rounds of therapy, which in this case would be three five-day treatments in the hospital with two weeks in between to recover. He forewarned me that it would be rough, but he was a little light on the details. It turns out that the treatment is so nasty that the typical person doesn't remember more than general impressions. I would have to live with the PICC line, and I thought I could make it through the treatments. I thought, incorrectly as it turned out, that if this guy could do seven treatments, I could do the three that I was scheduled for. Still, it was nice to meet someone who was living through it. Someone should have told me that I was talking to a guy with a very strong constitution.

I was also lucky to be able to talk to a colleague's sister-in-law who had been treated with Interleukin-2 for renal cell carcinoma. She gave me a lot of information about the treatment so I could anticipate some of the rather strange side effects of IL-2. This saved me from being freaked out when they happened to me. In case you are wondering, she is alive and well.

Despite my upcoming biochemotherapy, Virginia and I were scheduled to do the Los Angeles Marathon again. We had made commitments to donors who had pledged nearly $14,000 for our efforts. Virginia's hemoglobin levels were on the rise, but by this time she had only reached the count of 9.0. She was determined to do the marathon, and we asked Dr. Weber if I could do it with her before I began treatment. He agreed, but treatment would start three days after the marathon.

This marathon was very challenging. To begin with, it was one of those March days in Los Angeles when the temperature is in the high eighties. We both had the flu and though Virginia's counts were on the rise, 9.0 was very low. Then the start of the marathon was delayed for almost an hour by a post-9/11 bomb scare. Like thousands of other participants, Virginia needed to go to the bathroom after the hour's wait. After the start, she passed by the first four miles of portable toilets until she found one with a reasonable line. Even then she waited fifteen minutes. She claims today that her eyeballs were turning yellow by the time she relieved herself. Making things even harder, the marathon stayed on its pre-bomb-scare schedule. We worked hard to make up time, but Virginia got exhausted. I tried to pull her along by the arm, which only exhausted me as well. By the time we got to the half, the police were opening up the course to cars. The volunteers were shutting down the water stops. We continued, begging water from bystanders. At mile 20, the street sweepers were passing us and sprayed our shoes with dirty water. We reached the finish line in eight hours and forty-six minutes. It was dark, but our friends were still waiting for us, including my brother-in-law, Frank, and nephew Stephen, who had followed and filmed the adventure. Our friends and family would always be there for us.

March 6—three days before Van went in for his first round of treatment, we walked the L.A. Marathon again—very hot, very slow—blisters—finished in 8:46—raised almost $14,000. Feel good about that! But I think I'll retire from 26.2! It almost did me in.

The next day, Virginia had to stop Gleevec because of her low platelets. Would this ever end? What would this do to the progression of her disease?

In three days, I started the first round of treatment. It was going to be a very hard 2002.

7.

Biochemotherapy

Biochemotherapy consisted of a number of nasty drugs. It included two biological drugs (the bio part) that were there to stimulate the immune system so it could see and then kill the cancer cells. The first one, interferon, I knew quite well since it had been Virginia's first treatment; and I knew how bad that had been all by itself. I was assured that it would give me fevers during which I would probably shake uncontrollably and it would also make me throw up. I would get one shot a day for each five-day round.

The second biological drug was Interleukin-2, better known as IL-2. If there is anything nastier than interferon, it is IL-2. It would also cause fever, so if the interferon didn't make me shake uncontrollably, this would. The hospital would have cooling blankets and ice available, and they would give me Tylenol around the clock. IL-2 causes the face of every patient who takes it to turn beet red. It causes sleeplessness and restlessness twenty-four hours a day for as long as you take it. It usually causes a radical drop in blood pressure. Even though they would try to prevent it, there would likely be a great deal of water retention resulting in a weight gain of somewhere around fifteen pounds, so the staff would have to keep track of my liquid intake and outtake, which meant that I would have to pee into a measuring cup. There would be a good possibility for confusion and even hallucinations. Finally, there was some possibility that the liver would be affected and I could have heart palpitations. None of this would be enough to stop treatment. I would get one bag of IL-2 each day.

The chemo part of the treatment would start with Vinblastine. This drug was advertised as the most benign of the bunch. It could only give me numbness or tingling in the toes from which I probably would not recover. I would get five bags of Vinblastine each round.

Next was dacarbazine (DTIC), which is an old treatment for melanoma. It has been successful in extending life for some patients, so they throw that in as well. Its claim to fame is diarrhea. Dacarbazine also causes fevers, nausea, a suppression of marrow production, vomiting, hair loss, and suppression of appetite. I would get one bag of this drug every round of the treatment cycle.

The drug they described as the one that would bring most of the trouble is cisplatin. It causes extreme nausea and can shut down the kidneys completely. It can also cause hearing loss from which a patient is unlikely to recover. If the above drugs didn't cause me to lose my hair, this one would. I would get five bags of this drug per treatment. During treatment I would experience a drop in potassium and magnesium and there would be infusions of these as needed, and a constant flow of anti-nausea drugs as well.

The combination of these drugs could bring down my white count to the point where I would have virtually no ability to fight infection. To counteract this, I would go home with doses of Neupogen that would stimulate the marrow to recover and produce new white cells. The treatment team pretty well assumed that I could figure out how to inject the drug myself. There was some talk about oranges to practice on, but I had Virginia, who was by this time an expert.

I would go five days in the hospital and then have two weeks at home to recover. At home, Virginia would give me the Neupogen shot each day for ten days. She would also hydrate me once a day for five days through an IV connected to a bag of saline solution. I would arrive home feeling terrible, but as I got to the end of the two weeks I would feel better—just in time to receive the next round, which would likely make me feel a lot worse than the first. In all, three rounds were scheduled. Except for the Neupogen, all drugs and hydration would be delivered directly through the PICC line in my arm.

On March 6, 2002, three days after the L.A. Marathon, Virginia and I gathered up my underwear, pajama bottoms (so my behind would not hang out of the gowns), and sundries, and drove over to Norris Cancer Center. I had a short talk with Dr. Weber and then went off to get my PICC line installed by a nurse who was more friendly than proficient. She tried time and time again, but could not get the line snaked all the way through to my heart. Finally she gave up and handed me over to a physician, who tried to get it in while I was under a fluoroscope. He tried three times before he got it past whatever obstacle was there. This was an inauspicious start, and I would later pay for the snaking around in my vein.

The start of this treatment was a lot like waiting for the beginning of a marathon. I had to keep myself relaxed and focused on the positive. I had my drug pump, a square device mounted on a pole. On the bottom of the pole were wheels, and on the top was a series of hooks from which drugs and fluids would hang. The pump was a noisy little bugger when it was working right, pumping the medicine into my PICC line and then my heart. It was an alarm-filled little monster when disrupted. The decarbasine went into my PICC line first, and I didn't recognize much change. Next, I got my bag of Vinblastine, and then the cisplatin. Next they hung a slow drip of IL-2 that would take twenty-four hours to empty. Finally they gave me my interferon. "How do you feel?" "Fine." The truth was, I was beginning to feel pretty crummy and I decided to counteract it with a walk. Generally the pump runs on 110 AC, but it has a battery that allows patients to be moved to new locations without interrupting treatment or, if possible, to go to the bathroom or to get some exercise walking. I went for the walk in the hallway, all four bags hanging. I was trying to hide the fact that I felt crummy from those around me and to convince myself that I felt fine. Convincing myself that I felt OK was going to be a tall order.

That night, I found out what sleeplessness and restlessness meant. Not only was it impossible to sleep, but it was also impossible to concentrate on reading or even watching television. I am still amazed that I couldn't make sense of something as simple as television. Two things did make sense. One was the clock whose hands traveled unbelievably slowly. The second was the emptying bag of IL-2, which was the only bag left by nighttime. That bag would be my nemesis. I would watch it, looking for the slightest change in shape to mean that the volume of medicine had diminished. It seemed to change only when I slept, which wasn't very often. I continued to get up and walk the halls, a habit that would continue through the evenings of the first round of treatment. When I did fall asleep, I was constantly awakened for vital-sign checks and blood draws—or by the pump's alarm when my line got plugged, which happened at least three times a night.

By morning, I was pretty well through with the desire to eat. I was beginning to puff up, and my face was beet red. Though I was also getting very tired, I kept getting up to walk. It was that day when my view of endurance events changed from something recreational to something that had to be done to survive. My first event was a 5K, whose distance I plotted up and down and around the hospital corridors. I became a feature as I started and completed one event after another. I wasn't fast, but I did those 5K's pushing a hangar with my medicines swaying at every turn. I was trying to accomplish something, but the exact nature of what that was, was beginning to disappear in a world of confusion. A nurse friend would later tell me that walking is a sign they look for to identify a patient who is going to make it, which confirmed my new confrontational attitude toward endurance events.

One of the things the nurse told me before I started was that I might not, (meaning probably would not) remember much of what happened once the treatment took hold. This wasn't exactly true, but I don't remember a lot. I do remember the numerous walks—me, my pole, and the battery-powered pump. Once I went to the restaurant on the first floor just to prove that I could. I believe Virginia and I had a meal there. I remember tremendous kindness from the oncology nurses and Virginia's daily presence. It must have been hard for her. I also remember the fevers that were so bad that I shook all over with the chills.

On the fourth day I started throwing up, and that continued into the next day with a long series of dry heaves. After five days, on March 11, I was scheduled to go home, and I was ready. I had to empty my bag of IL-2, so I watched it like a hawk. Finally, that little plastic bag was flat with no more liquid to give it form. I had defeated that bag. I watched it die, but it was too late to leave. On Monday, day six, I was released and with that, found myself in a wheelchair and on my way down to the car and home.

Once home, we received a scheduled visit from a visiting nurse who brought me my very own pole for hanging medicine and a five-day supply of saline bags and all the paraphernalia needed to safely deliver their contents into my body. Tubing and alcohol swabs were included to keep all the connections clean. PICC lines are often the source of infections. Virginia would clean out my PICC line with heparin and then hook me up to one bag of saline a day for five days. Each bag was supposed to take four hours to empty.

My hair had been falling out all week, and by the time I was home it was pretty pathetic. I had seen this with Virginia and so decided to preempt my treatment-caused baldness by finishing it off myself. As soon as I got home, I called my nephews, Stephen and Craig, and they came over with electric hair clippers and buzzed me. It was at this time that I started asking for more hats.

Free from the hydration after the fifth day home, I went back to work. My puffiness was so pronounced that I had to reintroduce myself to most of my coworkers. I felt a lot better, but my mind just didn't function. I remember one very complicated piece of business that involved canceling a high-profile contract. A bright guy I worked with in the President's office, Jon Hagler, saw clearly that the combination of fog and fatigue was making me less astute than I should have been. He wrote a brilliant document for me that eliminated the possibility that others would see the difficult time I was having. I haven't seen Jon for a long time because he moved back East, but every now and then we exchange e-mails. Another friend I need to thank.

I developed a severe rash that no one could adequately explain. It was probably related to the Neupogen, but no one was quite sure.

I managed to accompany Virginia to UCLA for her three-month check up. Except for the demands my illness was putting on her, she was feeling great. The previous month's L.A. Marathon hadn't been much fun because of her anemia, but she was proud to have finished it, though she swore she would be a half-marathoner in the future. She had her blood tests, and we waited for the results. On March 25, Virginia's platelet count was high enough to allow her to go back on Gleevec. She had been off for three weeks. Progress, maybe.

Although I was feeling well enough to go to work, I had not nearly recovered when round two was to begin. On March 26 I returned to Norris. In went the interferon and dacarbazine then the Vinblastine and cisplatin. I began to throw up again. Next came the IL-2. This first dose of IL-2 was the strongest in the series and they told me that if I was going to have trouble, this would be the time. My face was redder than ever, and I continued to throw up long after my stomach was empty. This time I swelled up like a balloon and gained a full seventeen pounds of fluid in one day. For the first time I saw concern on the faces of my caregivers and they gave me Lasix, a diuretic, by IV, and I began peeing out the seventeen pounds. Still, I had to keep track of every drop. I had dry heaves all day on March 27, and my shakes had become violent. I tried to walk and made it down to the restaurant again, but that was it. I thought the dry heaves were too awful in the lunch room. Finally, I just curled up in the fetal position and waited for treatment to end. I didn't—no, I couldn't—talk to anyone.

March 27, 2002: Van is in Norris/USC Cancer Hospital undergoing a treatment called biochemotherapy. This consists of Interluken-2 twenty-four hours a day, interferon 10 million units every day, dicarbazine one day, cisplatin (four days), and Vinblastine (four days). He has to be in the hospital for five days and gets Neupogen shots for ten days.

He must go through three of these three-week cycles. This is all due to the 55 percent chance the lump on his head was metastatic. Three pathologists have looked at the slides, and they all equivocate. So to do everything he could possibly do, Van submitted to this. It breaks my heart to see what he has to go through. He's losing his hair, he has dry heaves, his skin is beet red, and his eyes are slits from all the chemo he's getting.

On the second day of the second cycle, he was shaking violently with the chills.

Virginia got her PCR test results and, for the first time, there was no evidence of disease. This meant that out of a million cells tested, no BCR-ABL was detected. The 600 mgs had done the trick. She had effectively won her battle, but she was so exhausted that it meant very little to her. At this time, I couldn't process the news very clearly.

I am angry that this is happening. My life will never be normal again. And my last FISH and quantitative PCR test came back 0 pH+ cells. With this going on with Van, my joy is dulled. I struggle to keep going, working, taking care of the dogs, driving back and forth to USC/ Norris every day, and living with physical, mental and spiritual exhaustion.

I did complete round two, but by the time I had, my kidneys were shot and I was technically at the point where I needed dialysis. My ANC, a measure of the number of neutrophils, which in turn is a measurement of the body's ability to fight infection, was 0, meaning that I had no neutrophils to count and no immune system to fight infection. I was severely anemic and pretty well destroyed both body and soul. I wanted to come back for round three, but Virginia and the doctor determined that it was over. Any more, and the treatment might kill me. I remember the physician's assistant, Monica Averia, whispering in my ear that I would understand why this was for the best after I felt better. No!!!! I thought I could do it again, but the obvious answer was that I couldn't. You can't will your kidneys to get better. On March 31, I went home very ill and very disappointed, and more than a little afraid. I had risked my life to save it, and the hell had been for naught.

It took me a while to feel like a human being again. Virginia still hydrated me through my PICC line, but the line was plugging up and hydration took five and a half hours instead of four. The next day we returned to Norris and a nurse was able to clear the line—quite a relief because the alternative would have been a new one. The next day I began to get my appetite back and asked for Virginia's homemade spaghetti. I sat down to my first civilized meal at home with Virginia in quite some time. Halfway through, I threw up back into the bowl. It was the end of lunch for us both. We next hooked up the hydration line. Joy of joys, it worked.

Finally Virginia convinced me to take Compazine for the nausea and it helped a lot. The rashes and the IL-2 redness began to disappear, but I began to blow blood out my nose. I continued to get hydrated and get my Neupogen shots.

On April 5 I had an appointment with Dr. Weber. My white count was .45, and my ANC was still zero. I still had no protection against infection. My platelets were down to 45, which explained the blood coming out of my nose. My hemoglobin was down to 10.9. Dr. Weber reemphasized that for me, the treatment was over. Anything more would probably kill me. Virginia and I were now happy to be through. I went home to my Neupogen and hydration, this time with two bags a day instead of one, eight hours instead of four.

I slept for most of the next three days. After that I went out for drives with Virginia, but returned home and crashed. On April 8 I ate a meatloaf sandwich without throwing up. In another milestone, the visiting nurse came to our house and pulled out the PICC line. I must say that it was about as creepy a feeling as I have ever had, but it was gone, and I felt good to be free of it. My hemoglobin would drop down to 9 before it turned around a few weeks later as the other counts began to rebound also.

For more than two months, I remained swollen and of course bald. My beard was gone as well. I was beginning to get used to having no one recognize me, and introducing myself to people I already knew became second nature. Sometimes I didn't bother.

My memory was impaired and my mental properties somewhat diminished. I went back to work and continued my supervision of the new building and initiated new international programs. I started to work out again, but I don't remember very much of it. I also went fishing with my nephew Craig.

On May 3, I had a CT scan and an MRI in preparation for my next visit with Dr. Weber. All scans were clear, and I was now scheduled to see Dr. Weber every three months and get rescanned every six months. Maybe my decision to go for aggressive treatment early in my disease would mean that I would be free from melanoma for the rest of my life. It would not be so, but at the time I began to feel much better and much more myself with the hope.

On May 11, Virginia, Tom and I joined with Virginia's best friend Judy Dunbridge in the Revlon Run/Walk for Women 5K run. Judy had been previously diagnosed with a virulent form of breast cancer. Tom and I machoed out and ran most of the race while Virginia kept her friend moving forward. The two of them had their pictures taken together as fellow survivors. It would be one of the last public things Judy could do. Though she lasted a while longer, she would die a grueling and painful death. Virginia picks her friends carefully and she loves them. Watching Judy suffer and eventually die would leave the latest scar on her soul.

May 19, 2002: Van completed two rounds of biochemotherapy, and then the doctor said enough. His kidneys took a dive (1.9—2.0 is when they do dialysis) his white count ANC was 0, he became anemic, and he was a sick puppy. Dr. Weber said since the therapy was supposed to be preventative, it would not be prudent to put him through one more round and kill him.

He is still recovering—gets tired more than usual, hair still gone, etc. Two weeks ago he had CT scans and an MRI, and everything is clear. Now he will see Weber every three months and have scans every six months.

Rosie is almost eleven months old and she's still a chewer full of energy. Annie seems a bit rejuvenated and seems to enjoy life.

May 11: Judy, my cousin Tom, Van, and I did the Revlon Run/Walk for Women's Cancer 5K. Judy and I had survivors' pictures taken, and Kenny Loggins performed in the Coliseum at the finish line. I raised $615 without even thinking about it.

Stephen did a really professional video of Van and me in the marathon. It's most impressive.

June 27, 2002: My little puppy is one year old today. How puppydom flew by. She looks a lot like Bonnie but still has her individual traits. Still acts like a puppy—chews, chews, chews! Races around and plays with Annie, who is very patient with her. Knows how to give "high fives" now—a natural arm motion like Bonnie's natural hugs. Rosie has found a place in our hearts.

On June 2, Tom and I did the San Diego Rock 'n' Roll Half Marathon. I remember standing at the start of the race and again having to introduce myself to my friends. My coaches were flabbergasted that I was even there. It was one of those races that is both challenging and invigorating—challenging because I was not really back to my healthy self. It took about half an hour of baby steps to get back to the car after the race. At the same time, it was invigorating as a sign that I was on my way back.

June 29, 2002: Another year of school over! If I live that long I plan to teach three more years. Then enjoy life.

On July 12, I had a checkup with Dr. Weber. I had been having a problem with the hearing in my left ear. It could have been caused by the cisplatin, so I thought I would mention it. It turned out to be a massive plug of wax. Dr. Weber had had a stint in a New York emergency room and among other things, had removed wax from quite a few ears. He claimed to have simultaneously removed wax and a cockroach from some fellow. He decided to take on my problem. He and Monica, using peroxide and warm water, did indeed restore my hearing. It wasn't quite a miracle, but I was grateful to about that level. The most important part of this process however, came when Monica said, "What is that dirt in the fold of your ear?" She then tried to rub it clean but to no avail. She had discovered what we believe today to be a regressed melanoma that was most likely the primary tumor that had started my melanoma experience.

On July 26 I had a biopsy of the regressed tumor in my ear. We would have to wait a few weeks for the results. But I was assuming it was probably going to be OK. If there had been any melanoma cells left in my ear, surely the biochemotherapy would have killed them. We had dinner with Judy to celebrate her birthday.

My appearance began to return to normal. My hair grew back on my head and my face. I kept working out and was feeling good.

August 6 was Virginia's five-year anniversary of her diagnosis with CML. She had survived her fatal disease. We needed to celebrate.

On this same day, I had the grand opening of the 52,000-square-foot Center for Training, Technology and Incubation. In conjunction with the U.S. Economic Development Administration, NASA, and state and local governments, we established the program as a model for business and job development. I was the master of ceremonies for the opening. The State Secretary of Trade and Commerce spoke, as did prominent officials from the U.S. Economic Development Administration. The event was topped off by a talk by Robert Parker, an astronaut and a representative of NASA. I was feeling pretty good and was anticipating the nice articles and photographs that were scheduled to appear in both the local paper and the *Los Angeles Times*. I knew I would probably get a raise for this accomplishment. I think this would be the point where I should have heard the Greeks in my ears talking about hubris.

After the hoopla, snacks and compliments, Virginia and I departed the grand opening for USC to keep an appointment with Dr. Weber. I have always liked Dr. Weber for his honesty and the way he is willing to think out loud, and this time he didn't disappoint. I showed him a couple of new bumps that I had discovered on my head that morning and he said, "Bad, bad, this is very bad." So much for delusion number whatever it was. He repeated that this could be nothing but bad and scheduled me for a needle biopsy thirty minutes later. In came a female doctor, one of a group of professionals at Norris who call themselves the Cyto Babes, pathologists who among other things administer and evaluate needle biopsies. She took the biopsy, then she and Dr. Weber went to take a look. Within two minutes, Dr. Weber came back announcing that he had clearly seen melanoma cells in the sample. He then said, "We need to restage you." Take my word for this; he was not talking about restaging me for the better.

At four thirty, I had an ultrasound of my right leg. I had previously had a blood clot in my left leg, and my right one was red and swollen like the other had been. Clots are not uncommon in chemotherapy recipients, but this time I was lucky. No clot.

At five o'clock, I had a CT scan of my chest, abdomen, and pelvis. The machine broke down in the middle of the test so they had to start over again and we were not out until six thirty.

At seven I had an MRI of the brain and we were finally out of Norris at eight thirty. We had dinner with my nephew Stephen and his dad, Frank and then arrived home at ten. The next morning I woke up to find my picture on the front page of the business section of the Los Angeles times. My work had been a celebrated success; Virginia was celebrating her survival milestone; and yet here I was, embarking on yet another battle with the unknown and unpredictable evil we'd come to know as cancer.

Still, we refused to dwell on it. We took off for Bridgeport in the Eastern Sierra where we have always found peace and comfort. We shared a charming motel on the Walker River with friends and family. As beautiful and peaceful as it was, Bridgeport and our companions there could not distract us from the fact we were anxious about the results of the ear biopsy and the scans. Even over the weekend, the lumps on my head were getting bigger.

August 9, 2002: Van's grand opening for CTTI was Tuesday, August 6—the five-year anniversary of my diagnosis. It was really a fine moment for him. Very impressive—The California Secretary of Trade and Commerce was there, as were NASA astronaut Robert Parker and top Economic Development Administration people—wow! Van was master of ceremonies for the event. I was so proud of him. The L.A. Times and Daily Bulletin wrote really nice articles on it. We were flying high. That afternoon we went to Norris for Dr. Weber to check a bump Van found on his head just below the other one. We were sent crashing down from flying high.

—Weber says "Let's do a needle aspiration."

—A woman MD comes in/does the needle biopsy/goes away to look at the cells.

—Weber comes in surprised and says, "These are definitely melanoma cells. I saw them clearly."

—"We will need to restage you."

—4:30 p.m. ultrasound of swollen, red leg that had blood clot.

—5p.m. CT scans of chest, abdomen and pelvis—machine breaks down as Van is in the machine. Out at 6:30 p.m.

—7 p.m. MRI of the brain/out at 8:30 p.m. Frank and Stephen, who've been at Northridge, join us.

—10 p.m. home.

Now I am at Virginia Lakes with Van, Ron and Betty Eaves, the Nelson family, and Van's cousin Bob. We were so looking forward to being here this year—new dog, and less pain than last year. But now, no matter how hard I try not to let it come in on me, I'm once again in pain in Bridgeport. It's hard to appreciate the full beauty here when your heart aches.

We now must wait for the results of all the tests, plus those from the two moles Van had taken off two weeks ago by Dr. Woodley. At the very least/best, he'll have to have more of his head removed. We are brokenhearted, and I'm very afraid.

We returned from Bridgeport on August 13 and we found that my scans were all clear, but the biopsy of my ear came back as "atypical cells." We had talked about removing the bumps on my head, but Dr. Weber finally said, "I cannot remove your entire scalp. We are going to have to do something else."

September 8, 2002: When we returned from Bridgeport on August 13, we found out Van's scans were all clear. We had an appointment with the surgeon on August 22. While in Bridgeport, the lump on Van's head got bigger and bigger. We were scared. The morning of the 22nd, the lump was imperceptible. The surgeon said he needed to call in Dr. Weber. Weber came in and they both scratched their heads. They decided Van should have a PET scan. He did and it turned out normal. Meanwhile biopsy results came back from a mole on his neck and a stain in the folds of his ear. The ear had "atypical" cells.

Appointment with Weber:

—Ear is probably primary tumor regressed. This theory a result of consult with several other people.

—Ear needs to be resected, wedge resection.

We are waiting for an appointment with the ENT surgeon for this procedure.

Today while I was sitting on the back patio, a bird flew into the bedroom window and fell to the ground stunned—Rosie promptly ran over and pinned it down. I pulled her off but it was badly hurt and could barely move. We left it there to recover, put the dogs in the house but forgot the dining room door was open and Rosie attacked again. Now the bird, still alive, is on the patio table covered for warmth while we wait to see what happens. It is heartbreaking. It feels like an omen. Who said birds portend the future?

On September 9 Virginia had an appointment with Dr. Sawyers at UCLA. Unfortunately her blood test showed a platelet count of 35 and she had to go off the drug. Her hemoglobin was only 9.1, but we were at the point where we considered that good news since it had been much lower. How Virginia was able to stand up to the stress and take care of me and the household with anemia as bad as it gets, is hard to explain. But something in her character keeps her standing straight under the worst of conditions. She has told me at times, "Van, you have to pull up your big girl panties and move ahead." I do my best with the underwear I have. By the end of the month, she was back on the drug. We got the PCR test results in a few weeks. It showed an increase in tumor load. It was none too soon to get her back on the drug.

September 12, 2002: BIRD UPDATE—The next morning it was rested enough to fly away—all better! What a relief.

I am weary—weary of so many things. Van's problems are taking a toll on me, and he is getting pretty cranky. I have to miss so much school for his medical stuff, and I have to worry, worry, worry. My heart breaks sometimes. Sometimes I am so angry that we have to shoulder this double load—me and him. I worry about my status too. I'm waiting right now for results of the last PCR and FISH tests.

Van has told me he has to travel quite a bit this year: Armenia in

October, Vietnam in December, Japan and China in April. I get so upset when I have to be alone, and he gets so mad at my reaction. I just keep wondering how much time we have together, and I am angry when I am robbed of that time. Van and I aren't talking very much right now because of this. The December trip means he can't go to the ASH Conference to find out the latest stuff about CML and Gleevec. I am so selfish, I am disappointed. At first he wouldn't be able to go with me to my next Sawyers appointment December 9, but Sawyers will be at ASH so I must reschedule the appointment. I cried when I thought he wouldn't be with me. What a baby I am.

This last year has been a tough time for me. When will relief come?

I have to go to an IB conference September 27-30 and have been feeling bad about leaving Van. Now I'm not feeling so bad.

On September 19, I had a half-dollar-sized piece of my ear removed and a graft from my neck fastened in its place. The surgeon, Dr. Dennis Crockett, muttered something about being related to Davy Crockett and that he was good with knives. This curious statement was on my mind as I went to sleep under anesthesia. I woke up with another little bolster stitched to the folds of my ear. He found no new melanoma in the piece he took out and theorized that it was all removed in the biopsy. On September 30, Dr. Crockett took out my stitches, and today my ear is as good as new. I am left to admire his work.

In early October I made a business trip to Armenia. Nice people, very poor country. This is where I learned that I could not drink with the Soviets (or ex-Soviets in this case).

On my return, Dr. Weber saw a big scab on my leg and asked me what had happened. I told him I had gone to Armenia and had gotten drunk in a drinking game that later caused me to fall out of a bus. He turned to Virginia and asked, "He is kidding, isn't he?" Her answer was that it was true and that she had no control over me. At this October appointment, Dr. Weber began to look for alternatives. I had two bumps on my head and he thought his best surgeon, Dr. Silberman, might be able to remove them and then I could get radiation to kill whatever cells might remain. He also began to investigate vaccine trials again.

October 13, 2002: Last FISH 1 percent PH+, Last PCR 7.5—very disconcerting.

Van had his ear resection on September 19. Had a tiny bolster like before on his ear because the surgeon, Dr. Crockett, took a graft from behind his ear. Now it looks really good—hard to tell he had surgery. Meanwhile, two lumps continue to appear just below the wide excision.

Rosie is such a puppy in grown schnauzer disguise. She still likes to nibble on your hands, chews off the tassels on Van's shoes, chews holes in her bed, runs around the yard like a free spirit, uncontrollably, and spends hours in the backyard if allowed.

She is so sweet and spunky. She and Annie get along very well, although Annie has to tolerate her spunkiness. Sometimes they chase each other up and down the hallway. They play-wrestle all the time.

It turned out that scans showed that I had more tumors on my head than I could feel, four all together. Dr. Silberman and Dr. Weber thought that surgery would be far too maiming. Furthermore, there were still no vaccine trials available for someone with my HLA type. My next adventure fighting cancer would be the CyberKnife.

8.

Cyberknife

CyberKnife is a form of focused radiation therapy. The machine that delivers it is basically an automobile-factory robot with a small linear accelerator at the end of its arm. With the patient on a table within reach of the robot, it focuses radiation at a specific tumor, but it avoids damaging surrounding cells by moving the beam of radiation around while all the time aiming at a specific spot. The only place to get a full dose is the specific location of a tumor. What makes CyberKnife unique over other delivery systems is that it can keep track of the movement of the patient so it can adjust its treatment protocol without stopping. It required the creation of a plastic mesh mask that would be bolted to the table to hold my head in place and still. In other forms of focused radiation treatments, I would have had a fixed device screwed to my skull; then it and my head would have been bolted to the treatment table.

On October 31, I returned to Norris to have my mask made. The waiting room was again full of brave people. Many of them were extraordinarily maimed by previous treatment, and I assumed that they were mostly at the end of their struggles. I then remembered that I was there for the same reason they were. That realization injected fear into my soul.

The technicians made my mask for the back of my head because they planned to treat me while I lay on my stomach. With the mask on, I had a CT scan and with the information from the scan, the physicist over the next few days designed a radiation protocol that had the machine delivering radiation to my head tumors from about every angle possible.

While we waited for my treatment, Virginia, Tom and I walked the Santa Barbara Half Marathon. We all had our best times. We had lunch at Cold Spring Tavern, a little place in the mountains we had frequented when we lived in Santa Barbara.

November 3, 2002: Yesterday Van, Tom, and I walked the Santa Barbara Half Marathon. Best time I've had in a half marathon—3:32. These walks are grueling.

Tomorrow, Van has to go to Norris Cancer Center to have radiation on the four lumps his head. They are using the "CyberKnife," which is like a robot radiation scalpel. He has one treatment tomorrow and one Tuesday, and that's supposed to be it. This is state-of-the-art treatment. It is as close as can be to getting only the bad cells.

It was around this time that Virginia began to develop a deeper involvement with The Leukemia & Lymphoma Society. She continued to do endurance events through Team in Training, but she also began to give presentations describing her experience of clinical trials and rescue, and the prominent role the LLS played in the development of Gleevec. Her first presentation was very good, and each succeeding one was better. She would become a regular speaker for the society.

On November 4, we returned to Norris to get my treatment. I should add that the machine at Norris was new and Doctor Zbigniew Petrovich and the staff had some things to learn. I have no complaints about my treatment and consider myself lucky to have gotten it, but on that day, they found out that with me on my stomach, the machine could not deliver from all the angles the protocol required because the arm found my body in the way. They were going to have to put me on my back. They made a new mask for me, gave me a new CT scan, and sent me home while they worked out the new protocol.

On November 6, I went in for my first real treatment. I got up on the table, and they lowered the mask over my head and bolted it down. I was given the usual instruction not to move. This was no small feat since the treatment was two hours long. It turned out to be an important instruction though because excessive movement made the machine hesitate and recalibrate before continuing and, of course, this would add additional time to the two hours. I was also told not to look. This too proved difficult.

After I was strapped in place and given instructions, everyone scurried from the room. I was all alone with a giant robot with a linear accelerator on the end of its arm. I closed my eyes, and the machine began to hum and buzz. I did OK. I coughed once, and sure enough everything had to recalibrate. I soon learned that you can hold back coughs and the need to scratch, but I was not able to hold back the need to look. In the middle of all the humming and buzzing, I took a peek and found a linear accelerator about a quarter of an inch from my face. It was obviously shooting radiation through my forehead at the tumors on the opposite side of my head. That scared the crap out of me, and I never peeked again.

I had my second and final treatment on the eighth. This time I actually fell asleep, which made the experience a lot better. I was grateful not to have snored, though. That would have stopped the machine. I got through it, but the treatment had a profound impact on my cognitive abilities. I was a long time coming back.

I dropped into a period where I was quite fearful about losing my job. All jobs are challenging, but mine was especially so. I was worried that if I appeared weak and affected by my experience, I would lose a job that I still valued, so when the President of Cal Poly asked me to accompany him to China and Vietnam, I agreed to go. Virginia didn't want me to go, but I did. I was out of the country for nine days. I had worked so hard to get and then keep my position that I didn't want to turn down the guy who controlled it. In reality, the trip had no purpose and I have absolutely no recollection of it, and worst of all, I had to skip the 2002 ASH conference to do it. It made me think maybe I needed some perspective on my professional life. I certainly needed to take more account of Virginia's feelings; after all, she had taken care of me during this miserable and trying year.

November 6, 2002: Monday the CyberKnife was having trouble. We finally got in for Van's noon appointment at 4 p.m. We got here an hour early, so this was a very long wait. Grueling, in fact. Van came back out in fifteen minutes. They discovered they'd have to treat him on his back instead of his stomach. No landmarks to line things up. So we came back yesterday for an 11 a.m. appointment for a new mask. This time the CT machine was down. Didn't get in until 1 p.m. Mask done—I had to scramble to get Lori Stephens to sub and to write lesson plans—go to Staples and photocopy handouts, give them to Judy to deliver—his appointment was at noon. He got in at 12:50 p.m. Treatment should be an hour, they said. Tomorrow he has his last treatment at 3 p.m. Then Friday he has CT scans and an appointment with Dr. Weber. A week at USC-Norris. Quite an experience.

I've had to cancel my hair appointment twice—once because of the marathon and once because of Van's appointments. Today I hope I can make my three forty-five appointment. I am suffering quite a lot of guilt about feeling upset about being out of school and worrying about my hair. I guess longing for a normal life is not unusual, but I still feel bad. Van has been really cranky—accusing me of making him feel like a zero. Like he isn't even there. He told me I was a detriment coming along with him. It was so stressful—made me feel even more guilty that I felt inconvenienced. I hope things will be better soon. My heart is breaking. I feel completely out of control and at the mercy of a capricious unpredictable force. And that doesn't even take into consideration my own situation. Wow!

Judy has been supportive as usual. She made a delicious chicken dish with salad and rolls, and Carol made brownies and ice cream. It is nice to feel supported. And Lori Stephen is subbing for me, which makes me feel secure that things will be OK when I return.

Somehow the realization that this is just the beginning is sinking in, and it fills me with despair.

Well......it's 2:50 p.m. and I'm still waiting for Van to come out. The one-hour treatment has turned into two hours and probably more. One more time. Cancel the hair appointment. Wow. Words fail me.

Thursday—no treatment—we went in at three, and at six they sent us home—the machine broke down. What about us?

Van did his final treatment Friday, November 8 and then went to see Weber.

I am supposed to be in Philadelphia today participating in a roundtable discussion about Gleevec with Brian Druker and five other patients. Unfortunately, the East Coast was assailed with a "killer" storm that shut down all the airports. Novartis cancelled the whole thing. I was very disappointed, but glad not to be stranded who-knows-where. The video press release they spent all day a week ago doing will still be released and aired on Monday.

December 8, 2002: This is the end of a very quiet weekend. Van is in Vietnam. He said he wanted to go to Philadelphia with me, but he felt he had to go to Vietnam with his boss to prove he could do such a thing (after his battle with melanoma). He's called a couple of times and today he said he wants to come home—only two more days for him—and me. I miss him so much when he is gone. Given our circumstances, I feel robbed of precious time together.

On December 13, I had a biopsy of a black spot on my head. It turned out to be a burn spot from the CyberKnife. By this time, I had lost a swath of hair on the back of my head where the bumps had been. At least I could see that the CyberKnife had been aimed correctly, and it appeared that the treatment had been a success.

On December 20, I had my appointment with Dr. Petrovich, who pronounced in a very self-satisfied way that the tumors were all gone. He called over Dr. Josef, the physicist who had designed the radiation pattern, and Dr. Josef insisted that I give him a high five.

Two days after Christmas, I returned to Norris with a very sore arm and neck and an ugly ripple on the left side of my chest. I was quickly admitted with a blood clot that went from my elbow to my neck. It was one last present from the PICC line that had been removed after biochemotherapy. I was immediately given an injectable blood thinner and then the oral blood thinner Coumadin, which I was told I would stay on for the rest of my life.

On December 29, 2002, I was released from the hospital and I went home. My leg still hurt and no matter what they said, it seemed like another blood clot to me.

On December 30, Virginia got the results of her most recent PCR test, which showed a miniscule amount of BCR-ABL. She had been on

Gleevec for the entire time between tests. Her platelets were holding, but her hemoglobin had fallen to 7.7. Dr. Sawyers took her off the drug again, but the hemoglobin reading would prove to be an error and the interruption of treatment was only a few days. Virginia's anemia would continue to force her to take breaks from Gleevec, but even then her PCR results would begin to stabilize at undetectable and nearly undetectable levels.

December 31, 2002: New Year's Eve. Yet another challenge. Van was hospitalized at Norris Friday and released Sunday because he had/ has a blood clot that goes from his elbow to his neck. Weber says it was probably caused by his PICC line. I remember how hard it was for them to get it in. Anyway, he's on Lovenox (the new injectable heparin) twice a day and Coumadin one more time. It seems my vacations from school are always taken up with stuff like this.

My test results show a FISH that is a little better and a PCR that's better than last time. Even though three months have passed, my platelets are holding in the 40s. But my hemoglobin was 7.7 yesterday. It's so frustrating. Since I want to stay on the drug, I have to decide what to do. What a drag.

The year 2002 had been one hell of a year, but as hard as it had been, we were both still alive, a triumph under our circumstances.

9.

A Try at Normalcy

Ambiguous at Best

For Virginia, 2002 had been a trying year and she had many nerve-racking health-related questions left unanswered. But not only did she need to keep herself strong, she had to take care of both me and her mother too. Her best friend Judy began a long slide toward death that was painful to experience. Virginia was held together by her incredible strength and her involvement with the people of The Leukemia & Lymphoma Society. It is fair to say that Virginia got through it partly because she found a way to give to others. Virginia continued to expand her role in the society. She became a regular speaker at Team in Training recruitment meetings. She was frequently asked to speak to newly diagnosed CML patients who learned, often for the first time, that they were going to be OK. She continued to raise money by running and walking endurance events through the Team in Training program, and she went to local schools to tell her story to kids who were fundraising for the Pennies for Patients program. Virginia believed that the LLS had saved her life by providing early support for the research that resulted in Gleevec, and her loyalty to the Society would remain unshaken.

The discovery of Gleevec and its remarkable impact on CML was monumental. It represented a paradigm switch that would lead to many other new drugs. On this subject, *The Washington Post* wrote a feature article that included Virginia's picture on the front page.

My problems eased up, but they were not gone by a long shot. I began to feel more bumps on my head. "Not good," Dr. Weber said again as he swung into action. On February 28, 2003, I had a needle biopsy of the bumps. Tests indicated they were not melanoma. I call this my year of false negatives. Over the years I learned to be skeptical of needle biopsies. Although these bumps were in a different spot on my head, they felt and looked just like the melanoma bumps I had in 2002. In March the bumps were still there, and I asked Dr. Weber to look at them again. Again he ordered a needle biopsy. This time the result indicated melanoma. On that day, I was sent to the PET scan center where they scanned my whole body. Something showed up in my gluteus minimus that had not been there before. Now we had to figure out what to do with melanoma on my head and something deep in my posterior. After an MRI, Dr. Weber called me and said this mass in my hip had to come out in order to find out what it was. He believed it was melanoma, but there was no way to find out for sure without taking it out. If this was melanoma that would mean that the tumors were no longer confined to my head but had spread to a distant location.

In early April, 2003 the president of Cal Poly and I again traveled to Japan and China. These trips were really beginning to drive Virginia to distraction.

April 29, 2003: I'm at the MRI place waiting for Van to come out. Tuesday of my spring break last week he had Weber check a lump he noticed a couple of weeks before—ANOTHER needle biopsy. Turned out to be melanoma. Had PET scan Friday of last week. Appointment today to discuss results and where to go from here. One week of intense anxiety—has it spread to organs, etc.? Results are negative except a place on his left buttocks. MRI is to confirm it is probably nothing.

This stuff won't leave us alone! It's making me so weary. Thank goodness my sub is my student teacher and Judy did the state testing in the a.m. with my class from hell—period 4. But it sure wreaks havoc on my professional life.

I am doing OK. My latest tests were pretty good—better than before. Miniscule amounts of PH+.

Went to UCLA April 24 to do an interview for the Healthology website. Met Dr. Shah who works in Sawyers' lab working on resistance.

He says they're beginning trials on four different agents. Very interesting!

April 30, 2003: While at the Arcadia TNT info meeting where I spoke, Dr. Weber called to tell Van (on his cell phone, no less) that the MRI showed a nodule that needs to come out because it could be melanoma. Surgeon appointment is next Thursday, May 8. We won't know if it is melanoma until it comes out and we get the pathology. If it is, this is very scary. It means it's no longer regional—these cells could be all over his body. Obvious conclusion: big trouble.

I'm devastated. I'm angry. I'm indignant that this could happen to such a wonderful soul who has such positive contributions to offer our world. I'm in despair when I think of losing my soul mate, my best friend. I wonder how I would go on.

This experience makes a person bone weary. The roller coaster ride is extreme and takes its toll. I can only repeat, "I am stronger than you. You cannot defeat me."

It turned out that Dr. Silberman was quite reticent to operate. He took me aside and said that "Dr. Weber is a very smart guy, but he is not a surgeon and doesn't always understand how difficult some operations can be." Operating on my hip was to be very challenging. The mass was right next to the bone. He wanted me to have another PET-CT scan, which I did on April 24. The test still showed a mass in my hip, but it didn't appear to be growing. Four days after the PET scan, I had an MRI of my rear end. The results were still inconclusive. The mass was indeed melanoma; it was just very difficult to prove. Dr. Silberman thought it was melanoma, but getting at it was so difficult that he wanted a positive needle biopsy before he would dig in.

May 11, 2003: Since I last wrote, Van has had his appointment with Silberman, who says he wants Van to have another (yet another) CT scan. Since Van is on Coumadin, he doesn't want to take him off it for a needle biopsy and then take him off again for surgery. He wants to make sure what he's dealing with. So next Friday he has the scan and the following Friday sees Silberman again. Meanwhile, he sees Petrovich this Tuesday about his head lump. This is a full-time endeavor for sure.

Saturday May 10. Van, Tom and I did the Revlon Run/Walk for Women along with 60,000 other folks. Once again, it was awesome. To see all the survivors and family and friends wearing their signs for whomever they're walking or running for is so touching and inspiring. I raised $450 for Judy and Shara and I'm proud.

Sometimes I feel like the world has cancer—but then I guess my world does.

On May 13, I met with Dr. Petrovich to make arrangements for another round of CyberKnife to get rid of the melanoma on my head. On May 16 I had new scans of my hip, and on May 22 I met with Dr. Silberman again. He still couldn't be sure and didn't want to operate until he was.

On May 29 and 30, I had my CyberKnife treatments. It gave me a burn swath on the back of my head, but the head tumors disappeared and I would never have another. Of course, I didn't know that at the time. What I did know was that this treatment left me a lot more mentally impaired than the earlier one. The day after, I found it difficult to process, and I am not sure how long this really lasted. I suspect at least a year.

June 1, 2003: Tom, Virginia, and I ran/walked the San Diego Rock 'n' Roll Half Marathon. Like the year before I was still swollen from the CyberKnife and had to introduce myself to friends. Tom and I were a few hundred yards ahead of Virginia at the 10K, but before we knew it she was running past us at full tilt. We came to a truce and crossed the finish line together.

In early June 2003, we learned that Dr. Blayney was leaving to take a position at the University of Michigan. It was a sad time because it is hard to let go of someone who has been in the trenches with you helping you fight death. Dr. Blayney would later be elected president of the American Society of Clinical Oncology. As fortunate as we had been to find a person of Dr. Blayney's talents, we were equally fortunate to find another good doctor in the same practice, Dr. Linda Bosserman, who was also willing to serve as an advisor for us.

Between June 11 and July 1, I had the two CT-assisted needle-assisted biopsies that missed the tumor in my hip and caused the radiologists to report that no tumors were there. Dr. Weber and I were skeptical, but since the second one had been done by the head of radiology, we accepted the conclusion. I was tired of CT scans and needle pokes, so I was certainly willing to forego any more. We left my hip alone for two years: Plenty of time for the tumor to grow.

Virginia and Judy had a good friend who, like Judy, had a virulent and advanced stage of breast cancer. On June 19, 2003, Shara died. At the request of her husband, Virginia gave the eulogy. At the family's request we would later adopt Shara's miniature poodle, Buddy. Then we had the fur children Annie, Rosie and Buddy.

June 29, 2003: Many things have transpired since I last wrote:

—Van discovers a new bump on the edge of wide excision.

—He has biopsy—it's melanoma.

—He has radiation (CyberKnife) on May 22, 23, or thereabouts.

—MRI shows nodule also. Surgeon (Silberman) wants to do a CT-guided needle biopsy.

—Results of this biopsy turn out only muscle cells.

—Silverman wants him to have another one because he doesn't think needle went into core of nodule.

—Appointment is made for July 1 (our thirty-sixth anniversary).

—I find out Blayney is leaving for a position as director of clinical studies at U of Michigan.

—Dr. Bosserman takes me as a patient.

—School ends June 20.

—June 19 Shara dies.

—I spend the Tuesday after school's out at her funeral, and I give a eulogy as her husband asked me to.

—Judy and I find out about her death at the last staff meeting of the year, and we huddle and sob next to each other.

—Judy tells me the chemo doesn't seem to be helping and the doctor must decide whether she stays in the study.

Last night we did the Relay for Life again. I bought luminarias for Shara, Judy, Rita, Aunt Phyllis, Van, and me. During the lighting ceremony, they talked about how the candles symbolized our lives and how fragile survivors' lives are, and how we are to go on in the face of that knowledge. It was depressing rather than inspiring.

Even though I was missing work during my different treatments, I could still do my job. I had a loyal team, and I had done my job long enough to succeed. I also think that what I had gone through had earned me some admiration from my colleagues and the president who had given me the raise I had anticipated, but I began to think about retirement. I had a terminal disease, and I was actually surprised I had survived as long as I had. In 2003 the goal was to extend this survival trend only. Certainly I wouldn't live that much longer. Virginia and I never complained, certainly never whined, and we enjoyed each other's company. Did we want work to interfere? We looked at our finances and discovered that we could retire if we wanted. We just had to decide if we should.

The fact was that Virginia and I wanted to spend more time together and work was interfering. My international travel, in particular, was causing Virginia a great deal of anxiety. Simply put, we didn't know how much time we would have together. Virginia was the poster child for Gleevec's effectiveness, but we kept to ourselves the fact that her life was still challenging. I remember one day when Virginia was scheduled to speak before the annual conference of Novartis's North American sales managers. The intent was to let the sales managers know that what they were doing made a difference to real people. The conference was in Century City and we had to park maybe two hundred yards from the front door of the meeting place. What no one knew was that Gleevec had driven Virginia's hemoglobin counts down to the high 7's. I helped her walk to the meeting, but we had to stop and rest in order to get there. Her talk was brilliant. She was on stage with Novartis's vice president of oncology, Deborah Dunsire, in front of a thousand people who saw her and Deborah projected onto a thirty-foot screen. I still haven't gotten used to the standing ovations like the one she received that day. Though Deborah is now president and CEO of another large pharmaceutical company, she remains Virginia's friend to this day. We had to stop twice getting back to the car. The anemia was becoming a long-term problem.

Besides Virginia's anemia, there were other uncertainties. Gleevec was a new drug, and no one knew what would happen in the long run. A number of people were showing resistance to the drug, and by this time Rita Rowbotham had died. The tests that measured levels of Virginia's CML were all ambiguous in these years. They often scared us. In July, Virginia's test was not as good as the previous one, and she started getting premature ventricular contractions (PVCs). Problems with thin skin began to intensify, and simple bruises and scrapes turned into ugly, painful wounds that were far worse than what a person with normal skin would experience. Every one of these wounds would leave a permanent scar. She began to get regular eye bleeds, which luckily didn't interfere with her sight, but attracted quite a few stares from people. She also got ophthalmic migraines, which did interfere with her sight. She would get wavy obstructions on the outer edges of her eyes that eventually converged on the center and then went away. What never went away was the edema, especially around the eyes. Don't misunderstand, Virginia was at all times grateful to be alive and healthy, but the real concern was whether these side effects of Gleevec would eventually cause real damage and if they meant that something was going terribly wrong.

Virginia continued to be interviewed on a regular basis, and she began speaking for The Leukemia & Lymphoma Society at a hectic pace. She had a way about her that made people cry without making them depressed. After all, her life and her experiences were triumphant.

Virginia and I were invited to serve on the Orange County Leukemia and Lymphoma Society Light the Night Committee. Orange County's Light the Night is a fundraising event that culminates in a 2-mile night walk around and through Angel Stadium, with everyone carrying a balloon with a small light inside. It was an honor to Virginia. She was also asked to be the honored patient for the affair. On August 5, 2003, a few months before the event, there was a kickoff Light the Night meeting of team captains, and Virginia was asked to speak. It was the beginning of a very special moment in our lives. Many of our friends volunteered to be team captains. One of them was one of

Virginia's former students, Lindsey Casper, an interminably upbeat and witty person.

July 20, 2003: Since I last wrote:

—Van's second needle biopsy is negative.

—Silberman is still dubious. Tells Van he can take it out and find out for sure (but it would be serious surgery) or he can wait and have another CT scan in October. Van decides to wait.

—I get latest results. FISH is 12 percent—very bad news.

—I begin getting PVCs the first week in July—still have them. Very uncomfortable.

—I get terrible hot flashes—I begin to wonder if they are menopause- or leukemia-related.

—Health Ed., a group that does education of doctors as well as patients, has interviewed me for a pamphlet on CML.

—I speak at fall season info meetings. I notice several people are crying. I wonder if my story will continue to be upbeat, or if I am once again in the fight of my life.

—I go to UCLA and have another PCR/FISH.

—Liz shows Dr. Sawyers an abstract from a meeting in Paris (Experimental Hematologist) that says that Procrit caused CML cells to resist Gleevec in the petri dish. Sawyers says it's poppycock.

—Van and I are on friend Maxine's Light the Night Committee. She asks me to be the honored adult patient for the affair.

August 7, 2003: Once again in Bridgeport. This time my heart is OK. Finally I can enjoy it here.

—I had a bone marrow test Monday 8/4. The worst pain so far and it still hurts when pushed on. (lying down, etc.) Liz and Sawyers are not worried about my numbers on PCR.

—Last results of PCR/FISH were 12 and 0 percent (second test). That's why Dr. Sawyers said I'd better come in for a BMB.

—Spoke as honored patient at Light the Night team captain kickoff. Lindsey Casper came—her legs and arms atrophied from not being able to move her joints, her skin scarred (brown patches, her hair peach fuzz). She was so lovely! Kim Patterson for Team Phissie's Fighters and Tom

Yeager for DBHS Leos were there. So was Keri Vigil, Judy Kerner's (Twiddler's) niece whose father died of leukemia a couple of years ago. I was so proud.

Lindsey was an elementary teacher who, like Virginia, had discovered that she had leukemia. Unlike Virginia, Lindsey had been young at diagnosis and had had a perfect match in her sister and so had opted to have a bone marrow transplant. But post transplant, she had had an extraordinarily challenging time. Bone marrow transplants are not a simple matter. The body can reject the marrow; the marrow can reject the body. The results are sometimes fatal, or as in Lindsey's case, debilitating. Lindsey's skin began to discolor, then thicken and then scar until she could not bend her arms at the elbow and it was almost impossible for her to walk. Her hair had mostly fallen out, never to reappear. But that didn't stop this young woman from getting on with her life. She married a fine young man and continued to teach elementary school. She still wrote on the blackboard; she just had to swivel at the shoulder.

At the meeting, in the middle of lunch, she told Virginia that she had a story for her. A few weeks before, she had been teaching her class, writing on the board, when a little boy screamed out, "Mrs. Casper! You are bending your elbow." Got to love those kids. Sure enough, for the first time in many years, Lindsey Casper was bending her elbow. She knew something good was going on. After the meeting, we watched as Lindsey hobbled to her car. Virginia could relate to how hard it was for her to do that. We looked forward to seeing her at Light the Night. Her plan was to walk a little bit of the two-mile course and then to be wheeled in a wheelchair to the finish.

On August 10, 2003 Virginia and I took our annual trek to Bridgeport and on August 12, despite Virginia's hemoglobin of 9.9 and altitudes exceeding 11,000 feet, Tom, Virginia and I undertook a nine-and-three-quarter-hour seventeen-mile hike from Virginia Lakes to Green Lakes. It was extraordinarily difficult, but it was also so beautiful that it approached a spiritual experience.

August 10, 2003: VIRGINIA LAKES TO GREEN LAKES:

—Tom, Van, and I did the walk yesterday.

—Left Virginia Lakes Trail Head at 9 a.m. and returned to Green Lakes Trail head at 6:45 p.m.

Virginia's strength still masked the fact that she had problems. Why did her anemia and low platelets persist? Why hadn't she reached consistent undetectable disease load? We didn't know and privately and honestly discussed the possibility that something was going terribly wrong.

On September 14, 2003, Virginia was asked to speak at a Leukemia & Lymphoma Society symposium where 14 researchers talked about their work. Virginia was paired with Dr. Shah, who was scheduled to talk about two patients, Virginia being one of them. We found out that the other patient was David Lawyer. We were introduced to his family, but before we could find him, Dr. Shah began his talk. Using a PowerPoint presentation and lots of photographs, he described the lives of both David and Virginia. Then as he shut down the computer, he said that these two patients had entered the clinical trial at exactly the same time but that unfortunately David Lawyer had died two months earlier. This is how we learned that David, Virginia's counterpart in the phase 1 trial, had not survived. Dr. Shah then asked Virginia to come up and speak. It took her a full thirty seconds to utter one word. As you might expect, Virginia pulled up her big girl panties and got on with the talk, but this event left its mark on both of us.

I think it was about this time that Dr. Shah rode a bike in Lance Armstrong's Tour of Hope. Virginia and Dr. Shah could compare the aches and pains of competition, and we still have a picture of him in his bicycling gear on our refrigerator.

September 14, 2003:

— BMB came out 3/20. No one seems too worried.

—School began smoothly. First period now begins at 8:01 a.m. but I still have to leave by 6:45 a.m. to have the time I need.

—Light the Night is next Sunday. Van's team at Cal Poly is eighteen people. Lindsey Casper/DBHS has thirty-one! So far, so good. Next weekend will be hellish. We have to fly to San Jose, drive to Santa Cruz

for Kristen's wedding, and then drive home because we miss the last flight. Then get up to return the car and go down to LLS in Santa Ana and be there all day and into the night. I'll be dead.

—Went for a retirement conference. Think this will be my last year of the routine.

—Went to an LLS/LA Chapter symposium where Dr. Shah spoke along with thirteen other researchers—reporting on their translational grants they got from the LLS—grants to translate what they do in the lab into the clinic to benefit patients. Donors and board members were there. I spoke after Dr. Shah. He gave a PowerPoint presentation of his work in the lab for the new drug for resistance to Gleevec. He also gave two case studies—on me with photos from babyhood to now, and of a man named David Lawyer who never got a cytogenetic response and died in July. The amazing thing is…

—He was 58 like me.

—He was in the history department when Van was at UCSB.

—His wife teaches at Crane Country Day School.

—He was the other patient inducted into the study with me in April 1999.

—He was a teacher.

I was overcome with emotion and almost couldn't give my speech. But I did. And researchers came up to me and thanked me for reminding them of the end goal of their endeavors.

On September 21, 2003, we all gathered for the Light the Night walk. Sure enough, Lindsey showed up and joined everyone with her lit balloon. We saw her in the crowd, lost her, and then we saw her again at the finish. To my dying day, I will not forget the moment when she walked up to Virginia and told her that she had walked the full route. In my mind beauty and spirit go hand in hand, and Lindsey Casper is definitely one of the world's beautiful people. She lifted our spirits with hers. And the event raised more than a million dollars for the LLS.

In early October, 2003 I went to Russia in support of a USAID program designed to initiate a tourism program at the University of

Petrozavodsk in the Republic of Karelia. I planned the trip so I could get there and back in four days.

This trip was especially hard for Virginia because the communication links were so poor. I had everyone in the hotel trying to help me make calls or getting hold of me if Virginia was able to get through to the hotel. These people were terrific. I remember having a drink in the bar below the hotel where the owner had commissioned a huge mural of the twin towers in memory of those lost in 9/11. This trip would end with an attempt to break the Republic of Karelia's record for the most toasts at one sitting, which was an amazing 174.25. The .25 was the result of complex rules that ensure that one of these bouts results in more drinks that the official total. I used my lessons from Armenia to survive this experience, during which we reached an astounding 84 toasts. I recognized the beautiful women of Petrozavodsk, the kindness of its people, and the new friends I had made. The last toast of the evening came from a person who knew what Virginia and I were going through. She recognized our courage and prayed for a good outcome.

October 5, 2003: Here on the patio looking at my beautiful impatiens and everything else that is thriving in the background, the balmy early October breeze caressing my being. I must admit all things seem right with the world. If Van weren't in Russia this week, it would be perfect.

Just finished the spring season info meetings for Team in Training (L.A. Marathon and New Orleans). Made a few people cry with my story—Marian, on our team for the Rock 'n' Roll Marathon and now a mentor, shared the story of her brother's death from lymphoma and shed a few tears. She's such a nice lady.

Looked at the photo on the wall of Van, me, Bonnie, and Freddie. Wondered how we can look so different now and how these two precious dogs can be gone.

My friend Judy is doing better. Her tumor markers are down to 100 (from over 200), meaning the chemo is working.

I'm getting more and more weary of the traffic on the way to school. Retirement looks good!

Van is in Petrozavodsk, Russia doing a job another person should be doing. Poor Van. It's such a long trip for only three days. But it will be cold as well as primitive there so it's just as well. The journey is from Los Angeles to London to Helsinki, where he'll stay overnight and then take a Russian plane to Petrozavadsk. Two days there, two days back.

I am off Gleevec now—for two and a half weeks. I wonder how many PH+ cells I have. Are they going rampant? I worry that when I go to see Dr. Sawyers, my PCR will be high because I've only been on the drug for four weeks or less.

I worry Van's plane will crash or that some other terrible thing will happen to him.

I wonder how I would go on without him.

By this time I had decided to retire, both from work and from hard drinking with Russians. I didn't think I would miss the day-to-day aspect of work, but I knew I would miss meeting and working with terrific people in exotic places.

On November 1, Virginia, Tom and I did the Santa Barbara Half Marathon again. Our times were good, but I got a blister the size of a silver dollar. We finished the experience with a traditional meal at Cold Spring Tavern.

November 9, 2003: Did the Santa Barbara Half Marathon November 1. Van got a blister the size of the ball of his foot.

Annie's kidneys started acting up last week. Wouldn't eat or drink. Now she's on anti-nausea meds and antibiotics and has had two fluid treatments. She's eating chicken and Caesar dog food but burps it up sometimes.

She looks so old—barely able to walk—and probably is pretty miserable. I'm afraid she's not going to be with us for too much longer.

Frankly I'm not ready for this again... It breaks my heart.

Status quo for Van. Hope and pray it continues.

Went to UCLA November 3. No results back yet. Sometimes I don't want to know. A new drug clinical trial began that day.

November 16, 2003: BUDDY COMES

—Annie is better after four days of hydration. Thank God for

Stephanie, who took her in and/or delivered her home. I know she is at the end, and it will probably be up and down.

—No news yet about my latest PCR/FISH tests.

-Took Buddy for photos at Home Pet Center/Furry Fotos today. He did really well.

Buddy is the miniature poodle we adopted. He's a cutie—black, as tall as Rosie, and as long as she is but weighs half as much as she does. He loves to lick and jump. We call him Buddy the Bouncing Boy. He is Shara's dog—only one year old.

November 23, 2003: My latest tests were more or less status quo.

Buddy and Rosie are already fast friends. They chase each other and play-wrestle. I'm so happy.

November 29, 2003: I am amazed that I am 58 years old, and I feel like I'm a child inside. I feel vulnerable and lacking wisdom—like I'm masquerading as a person who knows what she's doing.

The decision to retire at the end of the year is harder to make than I thought. It seems so final.

The next ASH conference was December 6-8, 2003. It was in San Diego, and Virginia and I went together. There were more than 400 CML presentations and publications in all. It was obvious that there was a lot of work being done on mutations, both on identifying them and on determining how to treat people who were resisting Gleevec. My cognitive abilities were not allowing me to process all of this as I once had. I was having enough trouble keeping up with my melanoma research. Virginia was so taken with the ASH conference that she too began to study her disease compulsively. She would soon become quite the expert and took over her role as the primary CML researcher in our family.

In a lot of ways, the conference was scary because there was so much talk about mutations, but little about the symptoms and problems Virginia was having. It wasn't a leap to wonder if Virginia might be facing more trouble in the near future.

On February 14, 2004, Virginia and I attended our first CML support group meeting. Computer-based discussion groups were my style. I mostly lurked and read and learned a lot. Joining a live group was more difficult. We had tried a generic leukemia and lymphoma group, and it had not worked out for us. We heard some very sad and scary stories from people with various diseases, and it was more disturbing than educational. But this one was disease-specific and supported by The Leukemia & Lymphoma Society, so Virginia wanted to go as a favor to a friend of hers in the Society. It turned out that this group was full of knowledgeable, helpful people who knew a lot that we didn't. We met people who were thriving on Gleevec, but most had side effects that compared to Virginia's and they had tried almost every way to deal with them. Some people were resistant and would be forced to change to second-generation inhibitors. Two more in the group would be forced into bone marrow transplants, and three others would die.

Though losing friends to the disease was very painful, we found this group helpful and upbeat. Virginia loved the group and subsequently would recruit a good number of new people who now adore her for it. Some of the participants were extremely knowledgeable about health insurance issues. They were able to help one of our members, Bonnie Dubeck, who had been dropped from her ten-year insurance policy after she started taking the very expensive Gleevec. And beyond the group's benefits to its members, it had raised more than $60,000 for the LLS.

April 23, 2004 was the night of my retirement dinner. My staff made sure it was top notch. All three presidents I had worked for attended, as did most of the people I had worked with. Reflecting on it, I think I had had an OK career.

May 9, 2004: News flash! Van officially retired as of yesterday (May 8). His retirement party was a lovely tribute to his effectiveness as a leader and visionary and friend. The loyalty of his staff was stunning. When asked what he'd like as a gift, he said a donation to The Leukemia & Lymphoma Society, so they presented us with a check for $1,000. It was very touching. At 4:45 p.m. yesterday, someone called and told him the governor had signed the golden handshake for CSU. So now he has to suspend his retirement for one day so he can get $5,000 more per year.

June 6, 2004: Annie still labors on. Many, many pee spots to clean up and bedding to wash. She can barely walk and we must coax her to eat. She has:

—Medicine for diarrhea.

—Medicine for nausea.

—Hydration two times a week. She falls over and gets lost in the cactus, behind the toilet, in the corner of the dryer, under the barbecue, etc.

Every time we think we must take her in to the vet for the last time, she rebounds and we can't bring ourselves to do it when she's perky.

Van got a blood clot in his right leg and can't do the marathon.

I'm sending in my retirement papers tomorrow.

Tomorrow begins the last week of school, my last week as a teacher.

Walnut Valley Educators Association had a retirement recognition for retirees last week.

Stacy Lind, Chris Buccola, Eleanor Reza, Sue Klinger, Irma Lujan, and others held a party in honor of the "Fabulous Five"—Judy and Bruce Dunbridge, me, Colleen Kelly, and Kim Cleveland—very nice.

When the school district heard about the WVEA thing, they slapped together a ceremony for retirees—they gave us four days' notice.

10.

Sorting Out Our New World

Preparing for the Final Act

I am conflicted about retiring. I will miss interacting with my students and learning from some of my colleagues—but that's all. Still, after 36 years of teaching and 53 years of going to school, it will be weird not to.

June 11, 2004: My last day as a gainfully employed teacher—a hard day. Gave away my files, video tapes, and audio tapes and walked out.

—When I got home, Annie was not doing well. Not any worse, but she hadn't eaten all day. Could hardly walk. We decided we couldn't make her go on.

—I called Sharman. Stephanie answered and told me to bring her down. I drove.

Van held her.

—When we got there, Stephanie was waiting with a towel at the door. She had tears in her eyes. She took us into Room 3—not an examination room. It had two chairs, a table, Kleenex, and lots of dog photo collages. Sharman came in and told us they would give Annie an injection of a strong sedative. It would take fifteen minutes to take effect.

—When Stephanie came back with little Annie, she was crying. So was I. Van held Annie as she slowly and gently slipped into slumber. I held her little paw.

—Then Sharman and Tia came in with the syringe filled with blue fluid. Sharman told us Stephanie had asked her if it would be unprofessional to cry. Sharman told her that it wouldn't be. Stephanie and I leaned on each other sobbing as they shaved a spot on Annie's leg and slipped the needle in. As the blue fluid went in, Annie softly slipped

away. She never even knew or felt anything. Safe in the arms of Van and with me holding her paw, she entered her next life. It was kind and gentle. Yet it was devastating even though it was merciful.

—I can never escape the emotional explosion that happens when I must do this final kindness for my dog. Waves of heartbreak drown me, and I feel like every cell in my body is being assaulted.

—The fine line between life and death is a most remarkable and fearsome passage to witness. It's a reminder that we all hang by a thread, and it brings deep sadness to me.

—Annie, pain in the neck that she was, was still my dog-child. I miss her.

I continued to think that something was wrong with my right leg and asked Dr. Weber to schedule another ultrasound. On May 24, I found out I had been right; this was my third blood clot.

Since I was sixteen years old I had been a pilot, and though I did not make my living from it, I flew often. I enjoyed what I could do with my little plane, and it was part of who I was. This third blood clot coupled with my metastatic melanoma made it impossible for me to pass a flight physical. This piece of me has been difficult to let go, and so I still refuse to sell the plane. I was offered a decent price once and I thought that Virginia would need the money if the melanoma killed me, but Virginia, sensing my thoughts, said, "Van you don't have to sell the plane. If you die, I'll sell it. You don't have to worry about it again." It was a relief to retain that connection to my past life.

Virginia had been training for months in anticipation of our first Alaska Marathon. Tom would be doing it with us, as would Tim Denman, one of my college roommates. My cousin Janet also signed up to walk the half marathon with Virginia. This was the marathon Dr. Silberman forbade me to do for fear I might dislodge a clot and die. I flew to Alaska to cheer Virginia and Janet on in the half and got carried away and did it with them. Tom did the full marathon and came in late with a young woman in tow. Despite finding her sitting in the dirt crying, Tom helped her find the will to finish. We followed the events with a week of travel—Tom, his wife, Tim, Virginia, Janet, and me. We had a great time.

August 3, 2004: Retiring has so far proved to be more challenging than expected. After Alaska, Mother began having falls. After two weeks of driving out and hauling her around in a wheelchair (if Van hadn't come, my elbows would be hamburger), a CT scan showed that she has had some small strokes. She is on several special care programs: incontinence care, two-hour checks, help with dressing, meals in her room, escort to meals, etc. Her rent has gone from $1,880 to $2,800 a month. She is better, but she hasn't come all the way back. Her mind is not all there. And as usual, she is depressed and whines all the time about it.

Anyway, today is really the first day I have had to do some introspection, and it has been a bit painful. As I got up to feed the dogs at 6 a.m., I thought of how three weeks from now I wouldn't be going back to DBHS, thought of how my name sign is probably coming off the door at this very moment, thought about how I will find some meaning in my life. Tears and fears reigned. I can see that what I thought all along–that this will be a difficult transition—is going to be true.

Van seems to have adjusted to his lack of high-powered activity quite easily. He has replaced his job as dean with investigating the Salton Sea and making a movie. He researches on the Web, reads and reads, and travels out there regularly. He doesn't seem one bit sad to have left his position. He is a bit cranky and short with me for reasons I can't figure out, and he criticizes me often for various things he thinks I am not handling right. So this part of the new experience is not working out very well. Even our tastes in television create unexpected division and animosity.

This morning when I shared with him how it finally hit me how different life would be, he replied, "If you want to dance, you have to be on the dance floor." When I asked him what he meant by that metaphor, he said that I am not taking any action to figure out what I will do next. He told me I have to get busy and do something—jump in with something and if I don't like it, I can always abandon it. This is the main difference in our temperaments. That is his style. It's not mine. I wish I knew what mine is, though.

I guess I need to mourn the loss I feel and move on. I do recognize the past is the past. But I still have regrets.

I also have déjà vu feelings about money. I feel reticent to spend money—worry about bills—worry about Van's charges on the credit card. I hate that. I thought it was in my past. I guess time will tell if my worries are justified.

August 25, 2004: I am sitting here at my computer sipping mocha coffee while my former colleagues are at DBHS having their first-day meeting finding out about the testing results from last year and probably rolling their eyes—I know I would be if I were there. It feels strange. I feel left out. I wonder how things have changed—the little things that make the routine of the day. I wonder how I will feel when school begins on August 30. It will be very different.

I have not made much progress on going through things in the house and getting rid of all the junk and organizing the rest. I did put an ad in the Courier for our couch. We will see if it sells. I have still not decided what my "niche" is, and I am still confused most of the time about what I want to do.

Our vacation to Bridgeport and Cambria went well. Rosie and Buddy had to learn to be good travelers. They want to bark and attack everything, and we spent a lot of our time trying to get them to be quiet. They also wanted to be on our laps in the car, which problem we solved by buying car seats for them.

Judy is not doing very well. She was taken off her clinical trial and put on Navelbene, which helped her chest lesions but allowed her liver and lung lesions to progress. So now she is on Carboplatin in addition to Navelbene and Herceptin. She goes for wound care every day for the hole in her chest, and she wears a pressure sleeve for the lymphedema in her left arm. It's a constant challenge for her each day, and she is stoically getting through it and remains positive. My heart is breaking. I feel so powerless.

Van and I are so happy we have little Buddy. He is such a sweet boy.

And of course we love our Rosie so much. We feel lucky to have our dog-children.

September 7, 2004: Well, another birthday passed on Saturday. I don't believe I ever knew for sure I would make it to age 59. I am so pleased with that. This morning I am sitting at my computer relaxing while my DBHS colleagues are teaching first period. I still feel a bit lost and hollow when I realize that, but it is a bittersweet feeling now because I do appreciate not having to go out at 6:50 a.m. and to be ready to be "on" by 8 a.m. It is nice to feel that I don't really have to "move" until I want to. On the other hand, I feel a bit guilty about that and don't like the idea of feeling "put out to pasture." Double-edged sword. I also wonder what my kids would have been like had I taught this year and wonder what fun interchanges I will be missing. It is best for now not to dwell on these things.

One of the best things about this new chapter of my life is not having to leave my dogs every morning. I know for a fact they like this too. It is a good life. I just hope we have enough money for me to do what I want to do and not feel like I have to be careful. We'll see.

On October 2, 2004, Virginia's good friend Judy died after a long struggle. By the time she died, the entire surface of her body from the waist up was covered with lesions. Virginia took care of her for the months before she died. Judy began to talk about wanting to be reincarnated as a dolphin. When asked why, she said then she could swim again and feel free. We all loved that woman. She was sweet even in her last days of misery. Virginia will never be the same.

October 24, 2004: Judy died on October 2, 2004. I haven't been able to write about it. I was there every day when she went into hospice. I helped with wound care every day. We brought her pillows for her swollen arms, sheet protectors, camisoles, Betadine, hydrogen peroxide, and sheets for her hospital bed. We were there to help with whatever was needed. I was with her when she died. Before that, I rubbed her feet, massaged her good arm to try and keep the fluid out of her tissues, and brushed her hair. I smoothed lotion on her feet and legs and got her some synthetic saliva and gum for her dry mouth. I cut her camisoles down the front and sewed on Velcro so she wouldn't have to hold her arms up in pain to get the camisole over the bandages. I patted her sweet face and told her I loved her. I kissed her goodbye each day when I left. The day she died I told her it was OK to go. After she died, the hospice nurse took out the morphine pump and neatened up the bed and took away the metal rack that kept the sheets off her feet. She lay there until the morticians came. Van helped them take her away. I felt like I'd been hit by a jet plane. I'm still trying to find all the pieces I shattered into.

Burial at Oak Park Cemetery October 5—just close family and friends.

Memorial service at Claremont Congregational Church October 7.

I am proud I could speak there of my love for her. Van stood behind me in case he had to take over reading.

The place was packed with people.

November 6, 2004: Our third Santa Barbara Half Marathon went well. Not my best time—3:43—but OK. More significantly, when we got to where the dolphins had accompanied us in the past, I scanned the ocean, though there were none to be seen. "Judy give me a sign," I thought. Still no dolphins. Then something made me turn around and look behind me—and there were two dolphins jumping out of the water and playing. Truly a mystical and stunning experience. Judy is having fun now and has made a new friend. She's not alone. I walked the next mile with tears streaming down my cheeks.

The new Bristol-Myers Squibb CML drug known as dasatinib was the topic of the day at the December 2004 ASH conference in San Diego. It targeted not only BCR/ABL but also SRC, a protein in CML's line of communication. It was advertised as 800 times more powerful than Gleevec and claimed to control all known mutations except for one. Again, Virginia and I went to the ASH meeting together, accompanied by our friends Roger and Nancy Klinkhart, whom we had met and trained with through the Team in Training program. Roger has chronic lymphocytic leukemia (CLL), and he and Nancy were as hungry for information as we were.

Dr. Sawyers sat next to Virginia at one of the presentations at the

ASH Conference. Dr. Shah said hello and gave her a big hug. Both Dr. Sawyers and Dr. Shah were playing lead roles in the development of dasatinib, and they delivered presentations about their findings. Clearly, it was effective against the vast majority of mutations. Would Virginia need it? We should ask at the next appointment.

When Virginia had her three-month appointment with Dr. Sawyers, she asked if this new drug might help her resolve her anemia and low platelet problems. He sensed our enthusiasm for clinical trials. After all, a phase 1 trial had saved Virginia's life. What he gave us was sage advice: Unless you need to, let someone else be the subject of a clinical trial. Let them discover the side effects. In the long run, dasatinib would prove a life saver for a good number of people, but it had side effects that were very scary for others.

In late December 2004, Virginia and I returned to Vietnam, this time not as part of a business trip but as tourists. Virginia and I had visited Vietnam together for the first time in 1994. Things had changed. There was development everywhere. We got to see a lot of our old friends.

December 22, 2004: It is 4 a.m. and I'm in the dining room wide awake. Bummer.

I can't get Judy out of my mind. I also think of Jodie and Sam, also dead from breast cancer. I wonder what was really going through Judy's mind during those last few months—whether she really knew in her heart she wouldn't make it. Especially during the last five months or so when her arm swelled up and her lesions got so bad. What a triumph for her to get up every day and tackle the everyday things (like getting dressed) that had turned into such challenges. She was so sweet and inspired such hope in all of us around her. I wish I could answer the phone one day and hear one more time, "Hello Virginia, this is your buddy calling." How I miss her.

I find myself wondering how long I will be OK, wondering how long both Van and I will be around. It is a strange feeling to think like that. I just want some time to enjoy Van and my dogs and my house and the world—a mindful enjoyment.

January 1, 2005: It is 4 a.m. and I cannot sleep. I don't know why.

Perhaps it is because I stretched out on the bed at 4 p.m. yesterday and slept until midnight. Why I don't know. Visions of Judy's last days are galloping around in my mind. Pictures of her raw chest, her swollen arm, and memories of her progressive debilitation each day she was in hospice. I can't get the images out of my head. I guess it is a delayed reaction. She was such a brave and sweet woman. I will always be angry that she had to go through what she did. I went to Judy's grave yesterday and put birds of paradise there. Someone had placed her ceramic otter and a little Christmas tree there as well as other flowers. I found myself sobbing because of the loss I feel. It is all so unfair.

Retired life is OK. Sometimes I feel a bit unproductive, but I am still feeling my way. Soon I will be helping launch a campaign of Pennies for Patients at DBHS. Hope it is successful.

From March 5-9, 2005, Virginia and I went to Baja California, to pet the whales. Sleeping in a tent camp, we spent most of the days in small skiffs, waiting for whales to approach. This was an intimate and almost spiritual experience with the world's largest animals. Mothers lifted their babies up beside the boats so we could stroke them. Some would move their heads right next to the boat, giving us an eye-to-eye experience as well. Others would display their athleticism with various jumps and other antics just a few feet away from the boat. We were glad to be alive, and it made us realize that we would not have had this experience together unless we had continued to fight. This made everything worthwhile.

After we returned from Mexico, Virginia took on some part-time work at her high school. She enjoyed going back, but by the time she was through, it was clear she didn't want to do it again.

May 13, 2005: I've been reading over my journal. Read through Van's struggle with melanoma and mine. Memories of the fear and anxiety came back. Juggling all those medical encounters with my job, taking care of Van, doing all the driving, and running things in the household—dark memories of dark times. The question of the future always looming. I realize how welded to one another Van and I are—especially me.

Some women always have to drive, always have to do the grocery shopping, always go places alone, always face fixing things around the house themselves. I've been really lucky to have a loyal husband for almost thirty-eight years now. Sometimes I take things too much for granted.

Tomorrow Van and Tom walk twenty miles. I'll do twelve since I'm only doing a half marathon. It's supposed to be in the nineties, so it will be miserable.

May 18, 2005: Well, I was certainly right about Saturday's training. It must have been ninety-five degrees or so, and it was pretty miserable! But it is over now.

Yesterday we went to the Salton Sea since I didn't have any tests to give at DBHS. We walked three miles down this sand-duney road in search of a deserted military base they used for bombing practice at the end of World War II. Van is researching the Sea and found out they test-dropped concrete-filled replicas of Little Boy (the bomb they dropped on Hiroshima) there. We had the dogs with us and there was no shade so the "pookers" got very hot. Plus, what asphalt there was on the road was very rough on their feet. But they had a very good time.

We came back through Julian and Ramona, a very interesting driving tour through Anza Borrego Park. I so enjoy spending such a day with my "guys"—all three of them.

In June 2005, we participated in our second Alaska Marathon. It rained, and I enjoyed it a lot more than expected. I like a rainy marathon unless the water gets into my shoes. The problem is that once you stop, hypothermia is a real possibility. The paramedics were busy that day. A woman collapsed on our bus trip back to our hotel. Virginia took charge, got the bus stopped, and phoned the paramedics to come and get the woman. For the event, Virginia and I raised $19,000 for the LLS.

In mid-August 2005, we returned to Bridgeport. We spent time with another old friend, John White, who had also been a college roommate. John has a four-wheel-drive vehicle and likes to drive it into the most remote spots imaginable. Together we saw the Eastern Sierra from an incredibly beautiful perspective.

Virginia's counts were going up and down, especially as she went on and off Gleevec. The fact was that she was OK, but no matter how many times her doctors told her that, we still worried —and rightly so. Errors were found in some of her tests, and they had to be done again with better results. Then, for some reason, Virginia's counts began to stabilize and her stays on the drug became longer and longer. By October 25, 2005, she was in her twenty-ninth week on Gleevec without a break. Her PCR test measured very low leukemia counts, and within six months her CML was undetectable. It was also becoming clear that if she were going to experience mutations, they would have already shown up.

October 25, 2005: I have been chosen for the Chairman's Citation Award from the national headquarters of The Leukemia & Lymphoma Society. They are flying me to Salt Lake City to receive it at a national volunteer conference. I am honored. I do what I do because I am committed to the cause, not for recognition, but it is nice to be recognized for my efforts.

I am in my twenty-ninth straight week of being on Gleevec—a record. We shall see what happens.

Last January I took up Ashtanga yoga and I love it. It is very hard and yet very relaxing when it's over. Very spiritual at the end, too.

Tom, Van, and I will do the Santa Barbara Half Marathon for the fourth time on November 5. We are ready.

Sometimes traditions are good and so on November 5, 2005, we did the Santa Barbara Half again. We again had our traditional lunch at Cold Springs Tavern.

On November 17, 2005, The Leukemia & Lymphoma Society flew Virginia to Salt Lake City to receive the Chairman's Citation Award for her volunteer activities for the society. This national award was a big deal and reflected how involved she had become in the society and how much she was appreciated.

Virginia took her friend Melanie Fastrup to UCLA in late November to see her physician Dr. Gary Schiller. Melanie had a rare and virulent form of lymphoma called Waldenstrom Macroglobulinemia. In the middle of the visit, Dr. Schiller blurted out that Dr. Sawyers was moving to Memorial Sloan-Kettering Cancer Center in New York and that Dr. Shah was moving to University of California Medical Center San Francisco. Virginia was devastated. The trouble when you find really good doctors is that they are often in demand. We had lost Dr. Blayney this way, and now we were losing Dr. Sawyers and Dr. Shah as well. Lucky for Virginia, this change coincided with the final containment of her disease, but she had other medical problems—most notably the anemia—that needed skilled attention. There is also an emotional attachment that develops between doctor and patient, especially if the circumstances are as extraordinary as those experienced by Dr. Sawyers and her. Was she going to fly to Sloan-Kettering to see Dr. Sawyers, or to San Francisco to see Dr. Shah? We thought seriously about doing one or the other. We also thought about going to City of Hope in Duarte, which was close to us. What we decided to do was turn to the last CML specialist at UCLA and see how we could relate to him. Luckily, we got an excellent clinician just when Virginia needed one. Within a few months, Dr. Ron Paquette had Virginia's anemia under control by adjusting the way she took Procrit.

The years 2004 and 2005 were relatively quiet for me. They were filled with intrusive tests, and though these were messengers of uncertainty, I was spared any scary diagnoses. All that changed on December 19, 2005, when my melanoma life got violently reactivated. A CT scan showed clearly that the tumor in my hip was larger. And in mid-February tests showed a new mass in my bowel. We were scheduled to go to New Zealand the next day. Dr. Weber said, "go," but that we'd be in for it when we returned.

11.

Slice and Dice and a Hip Full of Radiation

January 24, 2006: I am sitting in the waiting room waiting for Van to finish his PET-CT scan, Yes, we are back to that. On December 19, 2005, he had a CT scan (just a follow-up) and it showed that the nodule in his hip grew from 1.5 cm to 2.5 cm. Weber said it has to come out. Silberman was on vacation on December 23 when we saw Weber and got the news, so he couldn't be reached. We couldn't get an appointment until January 12 and when we saw him then, Silberman was not prepared—didn't even know why he was there. He needed to compare the December 19 CT scan with the other two done with needle biopsies and needed to talk to Weber about Van's Coumadin. It was really frustrating.

When he called Van five days later, he said he wanted Van to have a PET scan and another CT-assisted needle biopsy. This is all taking so long that at least they are letting us go on our trip to New Zealand February 16 to March 1, 2006. The nodule is way below all the gluteal muscles near the bone, so Silberman is concerned about locating it during surgery. I can't imagine what it will be like recovering.

On February 1, I had an endoscopy during which a doctor snaked a hose down my throat, through my stomach and into my small intestine. I don't need to add that this is not much fun. I remember being slightly under and noticing that someone had left a cupboard open containing quite an intimidating array of hoses. I wondered which one was mine. The results were negative, but only, as I found out later, because the tumor was in fact on the outside of my jejunum and therefore invisible from the inside.

February 1, 2006: I am sitting in the outpatient surgery waiting room waiting for Van to come out of the recovery room after having an endoscopy and biopsy of his duodenum. Last Friday, Dr. Weber called and told him the PET scan showed masses in his jejunum that needed to be biopsied. The report says, "consistent with metastatic disease or primary bowel tumor—stromal or carcinoid." At first his appointment for the endoscopy was next Friday, February 10; then Monday, they called and said the appointment was changed to today.

I went to the room with him, met Dr. Yang, and then he asked me to leave. I was just as glad to leave as stay—my stomach wasn't doing so well. I thought I was having a "Gleevec incident" but was determined to be with Van as he always had been with me for my bone marrow biopsies.

Now we wait to see what kind of cancer this is. What is in store for us? The reprieve we've had seems so short. I pray for another one. Van is such a kind and generous person with such a good soul. Why do these things happen to people like that?

I need to gear up for the battle ahead. I need to be strong.

I think Weber told Van that the hip thing is on hold because this new development in the bowel is much more pressing. I think he thinks this is very bad. And since the assistant came out and said they took three biopsies, I know there was obviously something to biopsy. And so we wait, wait to find out what our fate will be.

February 14, 2006: Well, Dr. Weber has us back at Norris today. This time for a test they call a "small bowel follow-through." Van has to swallow barium, and they take pictures as it goes through his bowel. It takes a different length of time for each individual. They said it could be three hours—or five—or six. We're supposed to go to lunch with Linda Abelman at one, but I don't think we'll make it. It's almost noon and Van isn't out yet. He began at eight thirty.

At 4 p.m. Dr. Weber wants to speak with us about the results.

I think I've figured out the reason for all of this. The endoscopy was for the spot in the duodenum referred to in the PET report. But there was also "a hypermetabolic soft tissue mass at the level of the pancreas likely reflecting metastatic disease." The CT scan says, "round 3.4 cm enlarged mesenteric lymph node surrounding the adjacent small bowel or an exophytic small bowel mass at the level of the pancreas."

The endoscopy ruled out a problem in the duodenum. Now we deal with the bowel/lymph node thing. Weber says it has to come out so we know what we're dealing with. This test today must be to see if this mass is "exophytic." I don't know what that means. Whatever the case, Van will be having surgery. Back to fear and dread, anxiety and uncertainty.

Is this what we've been hoping would never happen?

My reaction is strange. My anger is strong about this and it seems to be directed at Dr. Weber, who connects me to that which complicates my life now. I know one thing for sure—a good person like Van doesn't deserve this. That a person is good—or is making a contribution to the world, making it a better place—doesn't matter one bit to this cancer monster. Judy, Sharman, Shara, Van—-why? It is so ugly! Everything about it is ugly.

February 24, 2006: The doctors said we can go on our trip. So here we are in New Zealand while Silberman reviews all Van's tests. There are some conflicting things that he needs to resolve by talking to the pathologist, the GI guy, and by looking at the films himself. When we return, Van goes for another CT scan and an appointment with Silberman to find out the plan. Ugly—very ugly.

On March 8, I had a CT scan of my pelvis and chest. There was activity in both. Time for another needle biopsy. This time it would be the hip again. The hip biopsies had proven difficult, but a jejunum needle biopsy would have been very dangerous. If the hip was melanoma, we could assume that the jejunum was also. This time the doctors offered me an experimental PET/CT-guided needle biopsy. In fact, they recorded my procedure as part of a proposal to fund the project. Somewhere, a video of my bare butt is circulating among the researchers. I tried to read the radiologists. They see the tissue and they know, but there were no tells with these guys. Unfortunately, I made a good example of the need for the new procedure. This time they had hit the tumor and it was melanoma.

So, if the hip tumor was melanoma, then the jejunum had to be as well. My only option was to have both tumors removed. That or make plans for my demise. I was lucky to have a great surgeon, who was and is famous in the halls of Norris USC for his skills.

On March 29, Virginia's mother died. Taking care of her played havoc with our schedules and her habit of calling nurses horse's asses and the like was a challenge. But she was a part of our lives and her loss was traumatic, not to mention extraordinarily sad.

April 18, 2006: On Tuesday, March 21 at 3 a.m. Mother was taken to the hospital by the paramedics. She had slipped off the bed on her knees again trying to pick up the roll of toilet paper that had fallen to the floor. She pulled her cord and when they came, they asked her if she wanted the paramedics. She said yes. Then they came and since she had a bad cold, they took her to the hospital to be checked out.

When I called at 6 a.m., they said they were admitting her.

We drove to Hemet every day until she died on March 29 at 7:50 p.m. She couldn't fight off what deteriorated into pneumonia. The Saturday before she died, her speech deteriorated so that you couldn't understand her—it was gibberish.

Things just went downhill from there. The day she died, the lung specialist, Dr. Gupta, told me she was doing better. When I went in her room, I could tell that was not the case. I told her what he said and she said, "Oh for God's sake." Those were the last words she uttered. They were at 9 or 10 a.m.

While she could still communicate, she asked Van, "Am I dying?" He replied that he didn't know. "I don't want to die," she said, with characteristic tenacity.

Ultimately I think that is really how she felt and what kept her going. Despite her tortured existence, she didn't want to die. But the pneumonia was too strong, and she lacked the resources to fight it.

I miss her. She had a good heart.

On April 12, Dr. Silberman removed the two tumors. Having major surgery on your front and back at the same time is an unimaginable experience. I was cut open from my sternum to below my belly button, and I had a ten-inch incision on my backside as well. I woke up from surgery with my cuts, staples and a hose down my nose. The hose is called an NG tube, and it would remove fluids from my stomach until my digestive tract worked again. I poop and the NG tube gets pulled out, not one second sooner. In intensive care there was an old fellow on the other side of the curtain who pulled out his NG tube four times in one night. I learned then that there wasn't much point in freeing yourself like that because the nurses just jam it right back down your nose. I also learned from this gentleman's actions that threatening to sue does not work either.

The lessons learned from hearing my fellow neighbor struggle against authority made me a pretty good patient. One of the rewards was a resident teaching me that if you hold a pillow against your chest when you cough, the pain is greatly reduced and a nurse helping me figure out how to get into a position where I could sleep.

During the day, Virginia read to me the entire book *Ultramarathon Man* by Dean Karnazes, who ran fifty marathons in fifty states in fifty days. The reading was both soothing and inspiring. I remember at the time thinking, if this guy can do these things, I can get through this. I also remember thinking what a wonder it was that Virginia would read for me.

In spite of the fact that my literary mind was expanding, I wanted my hospital stay to be over. My main objective was the same as most patients in ICU who have had abdominal surgery—to go to the bathroom and get the tube out. Finally I farted and I began stripping down for a speed run to the bathroom. Then I pooped. Then out came the NG tube and all the IVs. Two days later I gathered up my things. I was liberated. Virginia took me home. Dr. Weber had told me that if I had the tumors removed, agreed to a course of radiation on my hip and had subsequent clean scans, I would qualify for a clinical trial of an experimental drug that might help me.

In June and July I had the thirty daily rounds of radiation. These treatments were inconvenient, but not very difficult compared to all I'd been through to date. I experienced a little fatigue and some burns, but I was able to take a few days off in late June to do our third Alaska

Marathon. It was one of my best marathon times and only reinforced my compulsion to do these races.

The radiation was followed by new scans and a meeting with Dr. Weber at which he told me my scans were clear, but that it was very likely that the cancer would come back. We knew that, and we had already agreed to enter the clinical trial for the investigational drug MDX 010. But the protocol required me to be clear of tumors so we needed to start the trial before something else showed up.

May 9, 2006: On April 12, 2006, two weeks after Mother died, Van and I got up at 4:30 a.m., left the house at five thirty and drove to Norris Cancer Center, arriving at six forty-five, the time at which he was to report to his blood test. However, the phlebotomy lab wasn't even open. So we went upstairs to the pre-surgery department. Thus began an odyssey that still unwinds today. I am typing this because I can't bear to write it all by hand, as laborious as it would be.

They had Van change into a hospital gown and lie on a gurney. He had to fill out forms, naturally. They hooked him up to an IV. It took a long time as he has difficult veins. (Five days prior to this, he went off of Coumadin and began injections of Lovenox—two a day since the drug store couldn't get the right dose of syringes. Weber wanted him to take 150 mgs, but the drug store couldn't get that in one syringe so he took 160 instead in two doses. They were very painful.) We waited in a cubicle while the nurse made various preparations.

Tom called at about 8 a.m. Said he and my sweet uncle Carl were coming to be with us and when should they come. When they arrived, Van was about to be wheeled to the CT scan room to get wires in his posterior where the surgery was to be performed and to receive the radioactive sugar that would help guide the doctors. When he returned at around eleven, the wires were jutting out of his backside and he was stuck lying on his stomach. He remained that way until noon or so when he was wheeled into the operating room. A resident introduced himself as Dr. Gupta, the anesthesiologist under the head anesthesiologist who would be doing the job. A woman came by and introduced herself as Dr. Nazarian, the surgical resident who would be in charge of Van's post-surgery care. Finally Dr. Silberman, the surgeon, came by and said the surgery would probably take around six hours. Van was clearly uncomfortable. As he was wheeled away, my stomach did flip flops.

Tom and Uncle Carl and I went to lunch at the Plaza Café there at Norris. I gave them my cell-phone number. Then the waiting began. They called me after three hours to tell me the hip part was done. Then at six thirty, Dr. Silberman came into the waiting room to tell me it was all over. He said the jejunum had clear margins. He said the hip bled a lot and they had to give Van two units of blood. He also said Van would be in recovery for an hour or so and then be taken upstairs to intensive care. I asked a few questions that Silberman, a man of few words, didn't really seem to want to answer, but he did.

Uncle Carl and Tom, loyal supporters, stuck it out with me and walked with me to the fourth floor where they told me Van was being taken. We waited in the waiting room outside the ICU and said hi to Van as he was wheeled by, drowsy, but awake. It was the change of shifts (between 7 and 8 p.m.) so we had to wait to go in to see Van. When we did, he had a tube down his nose into his stomach and several IVs in each arm. Some of them were for the monitoring machine; some of them were for pain killers, fluids, and antibiotics. Van seemed not to be in too much pain, just very sleepy. I kissed him goodbye, and we left to let him rest. It had been a very long day.

For the next six days I would drive to Norris every day, spend the day with Van, and drive home, arriving between 9 and 10 p.m. When I left each night, the walk to the parking structure was lonely and anxiety producing, but I always made it. And when I got home, my sweet little fur children gave me much needed comfort.

Since the McAndrews were in Hawaii, my dear cousin Nancy came over and took care of the dogs for me every day except for the twelfth when Stephanie from the vets came twice. Things didn't work out for having Stephanie the rest of the time because her work schedule was too problematic. I am so lucky to have such sweet relatives. Nancy was more than willing to help. Bless uncle Carl's and Tom's hearts, staying with *me all day, and giving Van hugs and kisses before they left. I don't know what would have happened to me if they hadn't been there.*

The first day in ICU I began to read Ultramarathon Man *by Dean Karnazes aloud to Van. We continued our reading sessions until we were finished with the book three days later. It is a very inspiring story, and it seemed to parallel what Van was going through and what I was going through vicariously and personally. Van tells people now that it helped get him through. His NG tube was the main problem because it would kick off a gag reflex when Van had to cough and then he would go into dry heaves. He couldn't sleep because when he dropped off, this would happen to him. One day when he got the dry heaves, my heart broke for him, but I was powerless to help. All of this was very painful and he kept a pillow close by to help make it less so. He endured this tube stoically for five days. He was out of ICU at the end of the second day, Friday. During the days he was in the regular room, he walked with his IV pole as much as he could. Uncle Carl and Tom came almost every day to see him, and one day we all walked downstairs and had lunch. Of course, Van couldn't because he still had his tube and wasn't eating. The tube sucked out the stomach juices so that they wouldn't irritate his stomach and he wouldn't be able to keep from throwing up. The stuff was ugly—dark brown, sometimes bloody. But it got lighter and lighter every day. By the time they took the tube out two days before he went home, it was clear. The doctors explained that while the intestine heals and is not working, the bile and stomach acids back up even though the digestive system is not being used, so the tube gets rid of that. When the stuff turns clear and isn't very much, it means the system is starting to work again.*

Van said he never had too much pain. Of course he was on major pain killers intravenously—two of them. When he got into his regular room, they took him off those and gave him a morphine button that he could press as needed every fifteen minutes, but I think he only pressed it two or three times. I admire his resolve. The Wednesday after getting into his regular room, Van went home. That night he went with me to walk with Tom and Letty, a longtime colleague and friend from Cal Poly.

It turned out that instead of walking, he took a nap in the car while we walked, and then had dinner with us.

This surgery was major for sure. Neither of us really understood how major. In a week's time after going home, we went in for a follow-up appointment with Silberman and they removed half of his staples. They left the others in because there was one place over the navel that was red, and Silberman wanted to make sure it was irritation from the staples, not infection. So he put Van on oral antibiotics for ten days. A week after this, the rest of the staples came out and Weber and Silberman agreed on a course of action that I detail below. This is the update I sent to all the people on Van's e-mail update list on May 5:

Tuesday Van got the rest of his staples taken out. He said he felt liberated! The surgeon and oncologist think he should have radiation on his hip since the tumor in his hip abutted some scar tissue right up against the bone. The radiation is a precaution to prevent recurrence in that area.

Yesterday we had an appointment with the radiation oncologist. Next week Van will have a CT scan (yes, yet another one) to establish exactly where the radiation will go—the surgeon left some clips there to delineate the area. The worst part of this is that Van will have to lie on his stomach for twenty minutes or so for the scan. It will be uncomfortable, but he thinks he can do it. If he can't, they have another way they can do the scan. Then when the scan is done, a radiation oncology team plans out exactly how to radiate the area without damaging organs such as the intestines and bladder. The type of radiation he is having is called IMRT—Intensity Modulated Radiation Therapy. This means they can vary the amount of radiation to different spots in the area. When this plan is done, we will know how many treatments, how often, etc., and then we will begin.

After the radiation is finished, Van's oncologist will put him in the new arm of his trial for a compound called MDX-010, which is an antibody to CTLA4, a protein implicated in the metastasis of several kinds of cancer, including melanoma. We are researching to verify that it is a monoclonal antibody. This compound is given as an infusion every eight weeks for a year. It sets off autoimmune stuff, so side effects include rash, gastrointestinal problems, and also in some people inhibition of the pituitary gland. They watch for these things and try to ameliorate them if they occur. So far most of the people in the existing trial have been helped—not all, but most.

Van is feeling better and better every day. Last week he walked twelve miles; once he did six miles all at one time! He has energy and now can sleep on both sides and get some good quality rest. He is the strongest person I know. He is my hero.

And so we beat on, boats against the current. Thank you all for your concern and support. It has helped us get through this challenging time much more than we can ever tell you.

Virginia

May 28, 2006: Thursday, May 25, we had an appointment with the radiation oncologist. When we first met him a couple of weeks ago, he seemed very nice. He is an animated, tall, muscular guy who is very disarming and enjoyable to hear talk.

Van had his CT scan, which they used to map out the route of the radiation beams. They put target marks on his hip with little bbs in the middle. A couple of days before we went in last Thursday, we got a letter from Blue Cross that they had denied the request for approval for the intense modulated radiation therapy (IMRT) Van was supposed to have. The letter said that the physician who reviewed the request said there is no proof that it is any better than regular radiation. This physician is a hematologist/oncologist, meaning she specializes in blood cancers! We were astounded. When I called Blue Cross and spoke with the nurse reviewer, she said that the doctor who reviewed the case wanted more information and requested that the physician call, but he never did, so since they have a time frame to approve such things, they denied it. The next day, we were to see the doctor. So I told her I would call her Thursday to let her know if we planned to appeal the decision. I had to call her the next day and tell her we would not.

When we got in to see the doctor, he took us into a room that had a computer displaying Van's CT scan from all directions and told us that

Van was to have eight weeks of standard radiation instead of three weeks of IMRT. He said when he saw the scan he realized this would be best. I said if he thought Van should have the IMRT, I felt certain I could get the decision overturned and he attacked. I mentioned that they told me they had asked him to call, and he said well, they are liars.

Van said that when we first met him it was obvious to him that this doctor was a guy who had a lot of buttons people could push. Van is sooo perceptive. I guess I pushed a button.

The previous Thursday, May 18, we asked when we would know about the radiation. They said everything was approved but the IMRT and that the plan was being made. I asked the nurse if they at least knew how many treatments it would be. He looked in Van's chart and saw the doctor had written down thirty. We were taken aback. We were told three weeks, twice a week. I explained this to the nurse. In the process of this discussion, I broke down and cried. I just had had it with being kept on a string and being called the day before and told to be at Norris for this or that—a pattern that had been going on since December. I mentioned to the nurse that I need information in advance in order to deal with these things and in order to schedule my life. (I have cancelled more appointments over the past five months than I can count on my fingers!) I don't think I am out of line to expect to know these things more than one day in advance. Anyway, apparently, the nurse relayed what had happened in this little conversation to the radiation oncologist, and he called Van and said he sure wanted to explain everything to him and especially to his wife.

I think he knew he screwed up and he got backed into a corner due to the fact that he now realizes he's dealing with intelligent people who take control of their health care. His reluctance to defend his position with the insurance company, or worse, his neglect to call them as they asked, was obvious to us. And for this, Van is punished by having eight weeks of radiation every day.

I really don't know what happened for certain. But I have been completely disillusioned by this experience. I have always felt Van was in such good hands at Norris. Now I wonder. I know that I don't deal well with people who feel that I should drop everything in my life to accommodate their poor planning.

I feel guilty that perhaps I am the cause of all this. If I hadn't broken down and expressed my feelings with the nurse, who then relayed it to the radiation oncologist, maybe he wouldn't have been so defensive—and maybe we would know what is really better for his radiation treatment. I am very low over this experience.

Van continues to get better every day. It is good to have him back. My life has been on hold it seems since January when the first stuff showed up on the scans. I don't know if my life will ever return to what it once was. I am profoundly sad that the melanoma has spread and devastated by the prospect of losing Van. I don't know what I would do. I don't think I could go on. Ironically, in the middle of all this, my last PCR test came back with undetectable cells. Hard to experience any joy. The last time it came back undetectable was when Van was in Norris for biochemotherapy. No joy then either. Also in the middle of all of this, Carol Veiga died of breast cancer and Andrew Farrand Jr. was admitted to Pomona Valley Hospital with a staph infection and a week later was declared brain-dead. They had to disconnect his respirator, and that was that. A really big shock. Death seems to surround me.

My profound sadness continues. It seems everything around me is falling apart. I would probably benefit from counseling but I feel too busy to find the best therapist. At any rate, now I can schedule my doctor's appointments that have been on hold and I MUST have several dental appointments for the tooth I broke when biting on a chicken bone in my chicken crepes Sunday morning at a restaurant. The tooth is unsalvageable and must be pulled. I'll have to have a bridge or an implant. And the @!# goes on.*

12.

Turn the T Cells Loose

June 15-18, 2006: Alaska Marathon: I'm actually writing this on the airplane home Sunday afternoon. The half marathon went well, although it was tough for me in what have become usual ways: I got blisters—a real doozie between my little and fourth toes on my left foot. My knee (left) acted up and by the end of the day felt like it was being stabbed with each step. Got a heat rash on my feet and lower legs, but not as severe as times previous. The hills were tough—and there were many, many hills. At least we didn't get rained on. Most of the time, the cloud cover kept us cool.

My walking coach, Kendall, stayed with me the entire time. She is so patient and kind. The half marathon course is tough for another reason—it makes participants feel like second-class citizens. Aid stations are few and far between, and there is no food at all—no oranges, bananas, pretzels, or other snacks. It's like they feel a half marathon is no big deal so we don't need any sustenance. All the resources go to the full marathon course—and they don't realize some of us are walkers.

I'm bummed out because I don't really think I could do a full marathon without damaging my body beyond common sense—even if I trained for it. With my low platelets, low hemoglobin and my PVCs, the results would probably be worse than when I do halfs. It is so depressing to realize I have physical limitations. But I do. Even doing a half does some damage.

Today I woke up with one eye a complete slit. I had to move my leg off the bed with my hands because it hurt so much. And the other leg with the skinned wound on my skin (from bumping into a pipe by the side gate Wednesday night) was throbbing. Then I had to listen to Tom, Van, and the other marathoners tell marathon stories including relaying all the various kinds of food they had. I was really bummed out. Van doesn't understand my daily small challenges with the side effects from Gleevec. I seem so healthy. But I'm beginning to wonder if I really am. At least at the moment I'm not dying of leukemia. I'm thankful for that. But I'm feeling a bit "whiney" about the other stuff.

Now we go back to our reality with Van going to radiation treatments every day. It's a harsh reality.

July 7, 2006: Van had his twenty-third radiation treatment today. He is supposed to have booster treatments. Yesterday the doctor said seven a week. Before that he had said ten. Van is supposed to go through another simulation before the booster treatments begin. Monday he was to go in for that, but after we got home they called and said to just come at his regular time—that he was having a treatment. He didn't ask what the deal is—new treatment plan? Boosters don't need simulation? Plan isn't done? We don't know.

This drives me utterly insane. I have no patience with this type of treatment—it seems disorganized and certainly doesn't keep the patient in mind. I'm starting to get used to it though, and now that I know their modus operandi, I'm not surprised at much of anything. It's just too bad I'm getting so disillusioned with this area of Norris after feeling so safe there and so well taken care of.

Tonight Van told me he went through his cameras and got rid of some that didn't work that he thought he might do something with—sell on eBay or fix—and it felt to him like he was settling his affairs—he didn't like that. It made him sad. It broke my heart to hear him talking like that. I pray he's around for a long, long time.

On July 14 I had an MRI of the brain and another CT scan, and all was clear. Although I had qualified for the trial, it had not been approved by July, so I had to wait a nerve-racking two months hoping nothing new would show up to prevent my participation. I worked out, with the trial always front of mind. Metastatic melanoma is a fatal disease. Scientists are still searching for ways to prolong life and even find cures, but they have largely been on an unsuccessful quest. Still, work goes on with researchers trying to get more out of traditional drugs, to make new target drugs work, and in the case of my doctor, to find a way to juice up a person's immune system so it can see melanoma as a foreign body and then kill it. The latter approach has a history of experiments with vaccines made in dozens of different ways but having in common a lack of significant results. However, in early 1996, James P. Allison, a researcher at U.C. Berkeley, published an article that convincingly explained the reason these early attempts to create vaccines failed was because CTLA-4 (Cytotoxic T lymphocyte antigen-4), a molecule on T-cells, was preventing the T-cells from seeing the cancer cells they were supposed to kill. He further suggested that a CTLA-4 antibody could be developed that would neutralize CTLA-4, allowing the T-cells to see cancer cells as the foreign bodies and then kill them.

Two companies, Medarex and Bristol Meyers Squibb, partnered with Allison to pursue the new approach. Together, they developed and started testing MDX-010, also named ipilimumab. In early trials it did exactly what Allison said it would, and the world of immunotherapy would never be the same. This was the world Dr. Weber was going to insert me into.

The problem with ipilimumab, though, is that if it works and does indeed inhibit CTLA-4, it gives the patient's immune system such a boost that it can and often does set off autoimmune responses such as rheumatoid arthritis, lupus, and very serious intestinal reactions that caused some poor fellow to lose his colon. At the very least, successful inhibition of CTLA-4 causes itching day and night.

None of this dissuaded me. I was six years into this disease, having gotten that far by putting up with a lot of slicing and dicing, a pot full of radiation, and a course of biochemotherapy whose effects pretty well defy description. I had new scars and the new nickname zipper belly because of the scars left by the scalpel and staples. I was statistically lucky to have lived as long as I had, but I wanted more time in what was and is a wonderful life. Since the scans showed no tumors left, I was eligible to sign up for the ipilimumab and the moment I could, I did.

Three days later, I received my first infusion of ipilimumab. It was supposed to take a while for the drug to take effect, so Virginia and I took off for a Mediterranean cruise. We promised our doctor that if need be, I would get on a plane and fly home. I must admit that I began to feel exhausted by the time this trip was over and once home, sunk into deep fatigue and began to itch the kind of itch that is hard to tolerate. Dr. Weber made me shave my beard so he could better see the rash that had developed on my face. Next I went into a high fever that lasted for weeks. My last real outing came when I went to a restaurant for dinner with my sister Connie, her family, and a dear cousin, all of whom have been a great support to us over the years. I rewarded their hospitality first by coughing my way through dinner and finally by rolling my eyes back and passing out in the restaurant and being hauled out on a gurney by the paramedics. I felt so ill that I had to cancel my participation in the Santa Barbara Half Marathon. Still, I was happy to see evidence that the drug was working and that the reaction didn't require the removal of my colon.

Two weeks later, I felt well enough to walk the Valley of Fire 10K in Nevada. I finished and was second in my age group but there were only three people in my group including Virginia's cousin, Tom. In his case, I tricked him by jumping ahead of him at the finish line. Virginia got first place in her group. I felt like I had completed a marathon, and I slept the 300 miles home.

During this time, Virginia began to see a rise in her hemoglobin. Normal hemoglobin for a healthy woman is around 12, but during the first five years of treatment for her leukemia, Virginia's was in the 8's, sometimes in the 7's. She did two marathons and three half marathons with this level of anemia. Procrit, the red blood cell stimulant, helped her some and brought the number up to 10. She did ten more half marathons at that level. I love to brag about her guts. Then, after years of struggle, her hemoglobin began to rise into the 11's. She began to feel like a normal human being again, and it was a good thing for me because I was going to need her help as my treatment progressed.

I got the second treatment on November 28. My fevers rose to 104 and I developed a persistent cough. On December 14, I had a study-mandated CT scan and its results showed something suspicious in some lymph nodes in my chest.

The end of 2006 was a year full of sorrow. Melanie Fastrup and Virginia had become fast friends and through that friendship, she and her husband Dan became involved in Team in Training—both as participants and when Melanie became co-honored teammate with Virginia. All throughout 2006, Melanie was able to hide her deteriorating health from her team until it was no longer possible. She had become chronically anemic and transfusion-dependent. Her doctor at UCLA was doing his best, first with Rituximab, a monoclonal antibody. When that failed to help her, he next began administering a drug called Velcade, one of the last lines of treatment available to someone with her disease. The situation called for a second opinion. Melanie and Dan knew of a Waldenstrom Macroglobulinemia expert at Dana Farber Cancer Center in Boston, but they didn't have the money to get there. The plight of this sweet woman and the desperation of her husband brought the team face to face with what cancer patients deal with on a daily basis. In October, one of our coaches, Katie McCollum, started collecting money from the team to send Melanie and Dan to Dana Farber. Tens, twenties, hundreds, frequent flyer miles, and in the blink of an eye the trip was paid for. We were all moved by what we had done and more moved by Dan and Melanie's gratitude. Dan wrote:

Dear TNT Family,

You all have become more than acquaintances. More than just friends. You all have become our extended family. We have been blessed by your love, concern and support. God has truly blessed us with each and every one of you.

Thank you for coming alongside of us in our time of need. We are so grateful that you have taken the time to find a cure for Melanie. As Melanie has had a setback in her treatment, we are going to Boston to see an oncologist guru who specializes in Waldenstrom Macroglobulimia Syndrome. We pray that we find a plan of attack to put her anemia in remission and keep her l gm (the B cell that keeps blood thick and causes problems when it is out of control) in check.

We want to thank all of you who dug down deep and made this trip to Boston possible for us. We will have more to say about you angels (messengers and ministers of God) and hope to thank you personally when we get back. Just know that you have given us hope and you have made a big difference to our family. You are truly brothers and sisters in the fight of our lives.

Melanie then wrote:

What is an Honored Teammate? Someone who inspires and motivates participants to raise funds for the cause. But something beyond that has happened here. You have become my inspiration to live and flourish, even with cancer! Each and every one of you has been there for me in different ways—physically, emotionally, spiritually, and financially. Because of you, I am encouraged beyond measure and have found new expectation. You have made the possibility of new treatment and cure a reality. I'm looking forward to seeing what God will do in Boston, and I thank you all for being His hands to guide us on this journey of life. We know we are not alone. Thank you for sending us to Boston.

See you at CHEERS…Where everyone knows your name.

On November 29, 2006, Melanie Fastrup died. At Dana Farber, she had learned that her doctor's treatment was exactly right. Under continued attentive supervision of her doctor at UCLA, Melanie continued taking Velcade. The careful supervision was essential because the drug had side effects that could be fatal if not for expert intervention, but Melanie had become tired of the long drive to UCLA and had decided to move her treatment to the City of Hope because it was closer to her home. Her friend and ours, Nancy Klinkhart, took her in for her first City of Hope treatment. As Nancy tells it, almost immediately after treatment Melanie began to get ill. This was unusual because it had not happened before. Since no one asked Melanie to stay, Nancy took her home.

Virginia knew that Melanie was home and decided to stop by to see how she was doing. She was worse. Her fever was up to 101.5. Virginia told Melanie that she needed to call the doctor. She told her that she already had and that she had been told to take Tylenol. Virginia helped

Melanie into bed and regretfully left. Dan was scheduled to be home in an hour.

About two hours later, Virginia got a call from Dan, who told her that Melanie was unconscious and in the middle of the floor; he didn't know what to do. Virginia told Dan to call the paramedics, and we immediately went to the house. Things were very bad. The fact was that Melanie was sick beyond retrieval. The next morning she died of Velcade-induced sepsis. Her family and around fifty Team in Training teammates were at her side. I remember the horror and deep sadness on the faces of all those present.

Melanie's death illustrates the inherent danger in taking these potent drugs. You have to be sure you have competent people administering them and monitoring their effects on you.

In seven months our friend Karla would lose her husband Scott to cancer. Scott was a spiritual guy who was studying for his doctorate at Fuller Seminary. Though these losses are the price of involvement, they are very hard to live through. Scott and Melanie were very religious people and though it was hard, their faith made things a lot easier. I wish it could be like that for me. And my fever and cough continued.

As I already mentioned, by this time I was fully involved with the ipilimumab trial. My life with the drug was difficult, but we would still try to do things. Our cruise was good, but after that I went downhill fast and was overcome by fevers, nausea, coughing fits, itching, and ambiguous scans. I tried to continue to walk, but when I couldn't do the November 2006 Santa Barbara Half Marathon, I had to face the fact of being forced to abandon a tradition that had helped me keep fighting. By December, I was so sick that we had to cancel our trip to the December 2006 ASH meeting in Atlanta. It was around this time that I began to try to train Virginia in the ins and outs of our finances. It was also around this time that I began to compulsively sort through my things. I was very sad once I realized I was settling my affairs.

November 1, 2006: The Friday after we returned from the cruise, Van got sick—cough, congestion in sinuses. Saturday he had a fever and has had one ever since. Wouldn't let me call the doctor.

—*Friday (one week after he got sick) he had an appointment with Weber for trial follow-up. We told the doctor about the fevers, but Van's temperature was normal at the time of the visit—Weber said his lungs were clear.*

—*Sunday. Fever went to 103 degrees. Tylenol brought it down.*

—*Monday at 11 a.m. when it got to 102.4, I put a call in to Weber, and he said to come right in for chest X-ray and labs.*

—*Chest X-ray normal. Labs normal. Weber takes blood cultures and gives Van Levaquin antibiotic just in case there is a bacterial infection somewhere. At six, Van takes Levaquin; he takes Coumadin at six thirty and then Tylenol for a fever that's back at seven fifteen. At the dinner table at Crocodile Café in Glendale with Jerry and Connie and Frank, Van has some sort of episode. He says he feels like he's going to pass out, turns ashen, and begins to tremble (arms and legs), then slumps over and does some sort of coughing/gagging, eyes glazed.*

—*Frank calls paramedics. Blood pressure low. By the time they get there, he's on the way back.*

—*They take him to Glendale Adventist emergency. They hydrate him and give him a CT scan of the abdomen.*

—*I had paged Weber and let Dr. Lieberman at Adventist talk to him. He agreed to some special blood tests—TSH and ACTH—one for thyroid, one for adrenal cortizone. Results won't be back for three days. Also more blood cultures.*

—*On the monitor all is normal—EKG normal, CT scan normal, labs normal—Van is feeling better.*

—*We go home after midnight.*

—*Tuesday morning fever returns.*

—*Consensus is Van was severely dehydrated—even though I'd been forcing fluids down him.*

—*Tuesday morning Weber calls, says to fax reports from last night and to keep him updated on Van by e-mail, which I do. Van's fever was bouncing up to 102 then down to normal or 99 all day.*

—*I made him drink 96 oz of Gatorade and eat as the papers we were given at Glendale Adventist said to do.*

—Now at 1 a.m. his fever is 103, and he is shaking from chills.

—I am so frightened. Weber thinks this is a reaction to the study drug. I just hope it's not something he got on our trip—the ship, the plane? If it is, we don't know it and he's not being treated for it.

—The fever thing is a lot like me on interferon. Maybe it IS the drug.

November 28, 2006: I'm in the day hospital at Norris sitting next to Van, who is in a chair hooked up to his second MDX-010 treatment. People all around me are submitting to the barbaric ritual. Sometimes all this overwhelms me and I sink into a funk. Then I feel guilty for acting ungrateful. I should be saying, "Bring it on—make Van sick—make our lives hard, but longer."

Van's problems continued until November 11, when the fevers stopped. After I last wrote he has developed:

—Mouth sores (bad, bad ones).

—Itches.

—Deafness in left ear.

—Rash on face.

—No appetite (Weber told him to EAT!).

The conclusion is it was a reaction to the study drug.

He felt pretty good for ten days—even did the Valley of Fire 10K—all uphill—and now here he is in for more.

Weber says the reaction will probably come sooner this time. I'm bracing myself for new fighting experiences.

Dealing with my emotions regarding Van's situation is becoming more and more difficult. My last PCR came back with a 2 log loss (.000081 to .0021) I am nervous about this being a signal of bad things happening because I haven't had to actually go off Gleevec for a couple of years. What happens if my own health collapses and Van needs me to help him get through the challenges? When I step back and look at us, I see how pathetic we are, how very sad we are as a twosome. How could this have happened to us? I don't even ask why anymore. For sure I get angry, very angry. And when I'm at Norris—the very place that is extending Van's life— sometimes I am repulsed. Although I know Norris helps him, I want to never go there ever again.

This last year has been so difficult. I've had to cancel my own appointments so many times. We canceled the Santa Barbara Half Marathon; and we canceled our registration, hotel, and our tickets to Orlando for the ASH conference. My life has revolved around what Van has to have. Surgery, radiation, CT scans, MRIs, infusions of the study drug, and nursing him when he gets sick from that.

I am angry and weary—-and add to that feeling guilty for feeling that way.

I guess this is what our lives will be from now on. I'm worried about Van. His cognitive abilities have been a bit compromised from all of this—kind of like I was on interferon. I hope he comes back. I hope this drug works. I dream of a life without cancer.

It will be strange not to go to ASH and hear the latest research—strange not to see Drs. Shah and Sawyers and Druker—not to say hello to the Novartis people. And not being connected to Dr. Sawyers, I don't know what will happen if I start having trouble. I am very scared. I am very anxious. I am very disappointed.

One day at a time…Sometimes lately that makes me weary too.

From September 29, 2006 through February 2007, my memory is a bit of a muddle. I know that I was taking the new drug and I know I was quite ill, but a lot of things are simply lost from my brain. I think some people minimize the mental impairments that come along with these powerful cancer treatments. This means among other things that there may be times when patients thought to be competent participants in their care are really not.

December 14, 2006: Well, 2006 continued to inflict its pain and despair. Melanie Fastrup up and died November 29. Since she had her first treatment at City of Hope November 28 and I couldn't take her (she asked me) because Van was having his second treatment at Norris, I stopped by the house to see her on my way to yoga class. She was very ill—throwing up in the bathroom. She had the shaking chills. I took her temperature. It was 101.2. Told her she should call her doctor. She said she had already called and the doctor said to take Tylenol, which she had already had done. I gave her a Compazine from the medicine cabinet, and she curled up on the couch. Her shaking stopped and she fell asleep. I left knowing she was resting easy and Dan was almost home. After yoga I called Dan, who said she was still pretty sick. I went home, fixed dinner, and ate. Dan called saying he'd found Melanie collapsed on the floor—couldn't move her—she was dead weight—wasn't thinking clearly—was panicked—what should he do? I told him to call 911, and Van and I got over there as fast as we could. Melanie was very sick and in bed. Then the paramedics came. She really couldn't answer their questions; she was unable to think.

At Pomona Valley Hospital, we waited for an hour, then they let me go in and see her. Her temperature upon our arrival was 105. Her kidneys were failing. She writhed on the gurney—said her back hurt, but really she could barely speak. The doctor said he'd spoken to City of Hope, and he doubted this had anything to do with the treatment. He said she might be septic. They admitted her to ICU. We went home.

At 6 a.m., Naomi, her niece, called. Melanie's organs were all failing. The situation was dire; they put her on a respirator. She called again at eight saying Melanie didn't have long before everything shut down. We went to the hospital, and I called as many Team in Training people as I could. We met Mel's family just outside the ICU in a conference room. They invited us to share some food. We went in to see Mel—she was unresponsive and on a respirator. I whispered in her ear who I was and that I loved her. She went on like that for three to four hours—her heart rate finally coming down from 150 to lower numbers each time I saw her. Finally it just stopped beating.

I was devastated, shocked, stunned. How could this happen so fast? Van did some research and found that Velcade can cause sepsis in some people and that an overdose can kill a person pretty fast. Should I have taken her to the hospital instead of going to yoga? I had figured she'd get through it and be better.

Melanie had had four other Velcade treatments at UCLA, and it seemed to be easier for her than the other treatments she had before. She even had gone back to work the week before she died. I will miss

Melanie so very much. She was always so positive, so supportive, so sweet. Another good guy gone.

By January 14, my fever was retreating some and I felt well enough to walk the 2007 Phoenix Half Marathon. This day turned out to be one of the coldest in the history of Phoenix; when we started, it was 28 degrees. I don't think this half marathon did me much good. I was getting some pain in my chest. I didn't tell anyone.

13.

It Wasn't Our Time to Die

On January 19, I had my third treatment. On February 2, another PET-CT scan examined what appeared to be problems on my December scans. By now I had bumps all up and down my arms. When Dr. Weber said he was 98 percent sure that the bumps were melanoma, I was pretty frightened. However, needle biopsies of some of the bumps were not conclusively melanoma. The people who do these biopsies usually don't tell you results directly, but they told me that the samples didn't look like melanoma. Dr. Weber told me the same thing a few minutes later, but he made it clear that he was skeptical about the results. Still, he decided to let me go through trial-mandated scans before he took me out of the trial and started giving me chemotherapy. I knew, and he knew I knew, that chemotherapy would have been the end of the game. Even though I had a hint of positive news, I was becoming very afraid. More and larger bumps and lumps developed in my arms and then around my knees, and some were as large as half dollars. They seemed to come overnight. In February I was due for my first Social Security check, but I didn't think I was going to make it. Still, I continued training for our fourth Alaska Marathon in June.

The results of the February 2 PET-CT showed lumps and bumps in my body–a lot of them—especially around my heart and lungs. This was when Dr. Weber said he was now 99 percent sure they were melanoma. I don't think I had ever felt much lower than I did at that moment. I demanded that he change the odds back to 98 percent. Honestly, this was the first time I thought death was eminent. It is not healthy to dwell on something like this, but circumstances shove the thoughts into your brain anyway. I was worrying about Virginia's finances if I died. I mustered the courage to talk to her about the accounts that comprise our modest portfolio. She wasn't interested because she didn't want to accept what I was doing and why. I wrote down what I could, and she filed it away. Thus began a flurry of activity getting my affairs in order. I went through papers, threw away stuff I had collected, and generally tried to tidy up my life.

January 19, 2007: Third treatment.

The melanoma monster reared its head again. After several weeks with no word regarding Van's CT scan in December (which we assumed was OK) Weber says (when I ask) he hasn't seen the final report—gets it—and says there are several suspicious spots—chest, hip, abdomen. They are lymph nodes, and he says the difference from the last scan is minimal. He has seen this before due to the immune system boost drug. He practically dismissed them and said they were not something to get excited about. Yet he ordered a PET-CT scan. Here we go again. Sometimes I wonder when Van will develop some other kind of cancer due to all the radiation from the scans and MRIs.

Van's appointment with Weber was at 8 a.m., so he had his blood drawn at seven. At ten, he still hadn't been called to the day hospital for his third treatment because the labs weren't back. Finally by ten forty he was connected up in some overflow area that had beds and a bunch of terse nurses.

Three hours for labs? Not bad, right! Now it is questionable that we will make our hair appointment in Upland at 2 p.m. and if we cancel, we sure won't be able to reschedule very easily with her tight schedule.

I am so tired of this. How many more appointments of all types—even my own doctor's appointments—have I cancelled in the past year? More than I can count. I'm tired of the way the medical profession thinks you have nothing to do but wait on them and their procedures. I hate this Norris place.

I hate this disease. I hate its relentlessness. I hate that I hate these things. I'm weary of living under a cloud of anxiety. But it's just too darn bad because no one cares.

Has this monster only given Van a couple of months?

January 29, 2007: I'm at the PET scan place, in the waiting room while Van is being scanned. It took this long to get the scan authorized and then to get an appointment.

The appointment was at 12:30 p.m. We got here forty-five minutes early, and they took him in right on time. At 2:30 p.m., after I had read the newspaper and a couple of magazines, and stamped and labeled 150 fundraising (for TNT) envelopes, right as I was beginning to anticipate Van coming out the door—a woman came out and said they hadn't even taken him in yet. Why!!? They had problems getting a vein for the contrast. Now why would that be? Because he has melanoma in his veins? I am expecting the worst from the report on this scan. I know Van is too. He hasn't said it, but I can tell. He was very anxious about this PET scan—I just read between the lines.

In a calmer state, I read the report again and noticed that there really aren't that many changes from the previous CT scan. There was one new "appears to be" nodule on the left base. And some "tiny nodules unaccounted for" in previous study. Then there is the tissue where he had surgery on his hip, which could be scar tissue or a recurrence.

I am grasping at anything that might not be so bad, I know that. I just want Van to be OK for a while longer. We need a reprieve.

As I sit here and the people who work here pass by as they go in and out of the office, I find them very irritating. I'm angry at their ignoring my suffering—at their indifference to my world cracking and about to shatter.

Ironically, I had my third-ever negative PCR report. The first was when Van was in the hospital for biochemotherapy: March of 2002. The second was when Van was in the hospital with his intestine/hip surgery (April 2006) and now this one, when we are facing major disease progression in January of 2007.

Thus we are robbed of the joy we could and should have felt at my recovery.

It is now 3:30 p.m., and Van still isn't finished.

February 28, 2007: Many, many more medical appointments since the PET scan! I note:

—*Weber telling us the nodes lit up and scheduling a needle biopsy (CT guided).*

—*Van not eating all morning, having blood drawn, us waiting thirty to forty minutes outside the CT scan room.*

—*Van hearing doctors talking in the hallway: "Garner's out there. Are you going to tell him? Not me." Weber calls and says pathologist says he can't safely do it—we go home.*

—*They want to give a consult appointment with a pulmonologist ten days later—I say no, too long—they get us in the next day.*

—*Pulmonologist evaluates films and says he can't safely do it either—the nodes are too close to the pulmonary artery and the aorta.*

—*Next day Weber calls the lung guy a "chicken weenie." Wants us to schedule a consult with a cardiothoracic surgeon.*

—*We see Dr. Robbin Cohen, the surgeon. Appointment is at twelve thirty. We get in at two thirty. He's very nice. Says the nodes are "underwhelming" to him. Shows us on the computer, thinks out loud. We like him.*

—*Surgery is scheduled for March 9 (Van wants to do the L.A. Marathon March 4) for mediastinoscopy and thoracoscopy. This entails regular surgery, small incision, scope down between the lungs in mediastinum, getting tissue sample.*

Van is having headaches every day. His blood pressure is very high too. He coughs a lot, but he always has.

The headaches worry me. I am up at 1 a.m. writing this because I can't sleep. Is the melanoma in his brain? Are the enlarged lymph nodes melanoma (as Weber says he is 99 percent sure of now)? How long does Van have?

I am sadly thinking about what it would be like to be without him. I am so sad most of the time, full of anxiety and stress. I know Van is too. He has told me how to keep up on our finances on the computer and has written stuff down for me. I am so bad at numbers and finances. I guess I'll have to overcome that.

I worry about Van doing the marathon with his headaches and

blood pressure. I can't force him to see the doctor. It's his life. I feel so alone.

In the meantime, I had been trying to prepare for the March 4 Los Angeles Marathon because I had made commitments to people I cared about, and not doing it seemed like giving up on the fight against melanoma. I was also afraid this might be my last chance to do a marathon. I managed one twenty-mile training walk that was extraordinarily difficult. I guess I should have heeded the warning.

On the day of the marathon, it was 90 degrees and I had a drug-induced fever of 100 degrees, but I proceeded anyway. It was part of a psychological battle with the disease that paralleled the physical battle. I was lucky to walk with two friends, Jacquie Ochoa Rossellini, who had walked the first marathon with us, and her sister Alex. Along the route we were not alone suffering in the heat and in response, firemen hooked up their hoses to hydrants and made these incredible waterfalls in the middle of the streets. I remember just standing under one ignoring my soaking shoes. Still, just before mile nineteen, I melted. I simply could no longer stand upright, let alone lift a foot. I had done lots of marathons and had never been defeated by one. I asked my companions to go on without me and with quite a bit of argument, they did. I was hauled to the finish line in an all-terrain vehicle. I will never forget the paramedic calling my number into race headquarters pulling me from the race. I was lucky to find my friend Terry at the finish line, and she helped me to the medical tent.

With the help of Virginia and Tom, I got home. I was stunned and petrified, but I didn't have much time to contemplate the events of that day. My goal was to stay in that trial.

I was lucky to have a doctor who didn't take his personal feelings about the tumors as gospel. He wanted definitive biopsies, but it proved daunting to find a doctor at USC Norris who would needle biopsy the tumors in my chest. This was irritating because the alternative was to cut me open in order to get the sample. Virginia calmed me down by explaining that these doctors did not have confidence that they could do what was being asked of them without hurting me.

March 4, 2007: L.A. Marathon Day.

I wonder if I've lost Van. Today between mile eighteen and nineteen, he couldn't go farther. The marathon folks took him to the finish line medical tent. No medal for him. He said he was leaning so far over he couldn't walk anymore. Jacquie Ochoa Rossellini tried to help him like I did, but to no avail. At the medical tent, I saw his papers they filled out—BP 130/80, pulse 88. We walked to the train station. Van swayed and gingerly walked. Stairs were scary. But we got to Union Station, and Tom took us to the Madre Gold Line Station, and I drove home.

Now Van has a temp of 100.9. I pray I won't have to take him to the emergency room or to Norris.

March 9, 2007: Van was supposed to have the surgical biopsy today. However, late yesterday afternoon, the doctor's office called and told Van the surgery was postponed to Tuesday (the thirteenth) due to his blood being too thin. (Of course his blood test was given before he stopped Coumadin.) We are both right on the edge. Van has severe troublesome symptoms!

—Couldn't finish his meals.

—Cold all the time.

—Low-grade fever.

—Fatigue.

—Depressed.

I am struggling, but I go on.

March was the month during which Virginia and I were becoming quite aware that I might die. I was riddled with bumps and lumps that everyone thought were melanoma.

Finally, a week after the L.A. Marathon, I had surgery to biopsy the internal tumors. A very experienced doctor went through an incision in my neck and then three between my ribs. I found out, firsthand, what kind of surgery Dr. Weber was trying to protect me from. The samples went to the lab while I was still under and, much to everyone's surprise, it turned out that none were melanoma. They were sarcoid granulomas, the result of a ipilimumab-induced autoimmune reaction called sarcoidosis. Ipilimumab gave us perverse signs that it had worked.

Still, it took a nasty surgery to find this out and sarcoidosis has a very nasty impact on the body, but it does not usually kill. I won't ever forget the surgeon when he came to me beaming and said, "I could never imagine being happy to tell someone that they had sarcoidosis." The sarcoidosis was a reaction of the type that had been seen in only one other trial participant. The drug was working, and I still had my colon. I still had fevers and various drains, felt terrible, and was very sore from the surgery. My kidneys were completely out of whack because I had been given an incorrect drug for pain, but I was not scheduled to die. This time Virginia would read to me John Bingham's book, *The Courage to Start*. A few days later I returned home. Virginia drove me to practice that weekend, though I only managed a few miles.

After the February/March nightmare, I did all I could to look healthy so Dr. Weber, Medarex, Bristol-Myers-Squibb, and the FDA would approve me for a fourth treatment. I had blood tests, lung tests, and a biopsy of a new bump on my knee. It too was sarcoidosis. The sarcoidosis side effects intensified. My weight dropped ten pounds. Still, when asked how I felt, I always said I was fine. I came to talk about the L.A. Marathon as if it were a victory and evidence of that fact. I wanted that fourth treatment.

I thought I had made it and showed up on treatment day with my reading materials and my snacks. I got as far as getting my blood tests done before Dr. Weber caught up with me and told me that the treatments were over for me. He told me that I had had such a strong reaction to the drug that another infusion might intensify the reaction to the point where it might do me irretrievable harm. After everything I had done to get to the fourth treatment, I was devastated. After all this, I was still going to die! I must not have hidden my thoughts very well because Dr. Weber then looked me in the eye and told me that he had only seen a very few people with responses of my intensity and that none of them had relapsed and that I wasn't going to either. Further treatments were pointless because all evidence showed that one major reaction was all that was needed. Technically I would remain in the trial, because I had become a "person of interest" because the sarcoids were so unusual, but

I was being removed from actual treatment. After I calmed down a little, I decided that I would try to believe the doctor that I would not relapse. Besides, I didn't want to join the guy without a colon, and I didn't want to be the first person killed by this treatment. I was going to live, not die. Best to leave it like that.

April 11, 2007: It has been a month since Van's surgical biopsy of the enlarged lymph nodes in his chest and the unfortunate event of his kidneys crashing. He is better, but still not back to how he was before all this happened. With normal creatinine being 1.4, his is 1.5, or it was a week and a half ago. He is back to walking every day, sleeping during the day less, and eating more. Still has to drink eight glasses of water a day, and it is killing him. I can't imagine that his body has withstood all it has in the past few years, especially this past year. I can't imagine how it can ever get back to normal.

As caregiver, I find it challenging to live with all the medical appointments and the aberrant behavior, but I am glad I can be there for Van just like he was there for me. Sometimes, though, my anxiety level goes over the top, and I worry about my own health and what this will do to it. Hopefully, I will be strong enough to endure and overcome.

Van is truly a man of courage, and I admire him so much. Sometimes though, he doesn't exercise common sense in taking care of himself, and there is nothing I can do and that is frustrating. I think he pushed it too hard last night at hill training, and he spent the day sleeping. He had a coughing fit that led to gagging and vomiting, and that is very distressing to witness—and I am sure for him to experience, too. I pray for even better days for him.

April 24, 2007: Well, we are now separated from that nightmare and I am glad. To catch up:

—Van had a mediastinoscopy (incision at collar bone and under sternum) and a thoracoscopy (three incisions on right chest) on March 13. I wasn't happy about the thirteenth thing, but it turned out OK.

—Letty and Tom came at 5:30 a.m. to be with us before the surgery. It was comforting. Letty then went to work.

—When Tom and I got to the waiting room, Terri Engler was there.

She was to stay with me until Van was taken to his room at 4 p.m., bless her heart.

—Dr. Cohen came at about 10 a.m. or so to tell me that the lymph nodes were not enlarged with melanoma, but rather that the enlargement was caused by "caseating granulomas," the hallmark of sarcoidosis (an autoimmune disorder). He was actually joyful and said he couldn't believe he was so happy about telling a patient's family they have sarcoidosis. Tom was there. I burst into tears, and he held me and let me cry. Dr. Cohen was touched, I could tell. Tom was emotional, too.

—Van was in the hospital for three days. He had a chest tube for the first two. They left his epidural in (for pain) until the day he left, and it is now thought that his kidney failure (creatinine 2.9—normal 1.3) might have been caused by the painkiller they gave him through it. It actually took a month for his creatinine to go down to 1.4.

—Since then we've been going to one doctor or another—two to three times a week. Because of the sarcoidosis, Weber and the drug company, Bristol-Myers Squibb, are most interested in Van. It turns out he's one of only two people in the world who have taken MDX-010 to get sarcoidosis, They want to follow him and keep him on the drug, but are putting him through various "stuff" before they allow him to have the next treatment in three weeks. So far he's:

—Had a breathing test (it came out well).

—Now taking a beta blocker for his blood pressure.

—Seen a pulmonologist who is making him have his eyes checked for sarcoidosis.

—Has been drinking voluminous amounts of liquids for his kidneys.

—Had a biopsy of bumps that appeared above his knee (they're negative).

I'm waiting at the PET imaging place. This time there's a nice lady behind the desk—oh—Van just came out. It only took two hours and forty minutes this time!

And by the way I just got my March PCR results—no detectable leukemia cells! Van seems to be doing pretty well. He's frustrated, though, because Silberman won't let him "train" until the stitches are out of his knee on May 10.

Van does admit he's pretty tired. That's one of the side effects of the blood pressure drug he's taking. He also has some cognitive problems—memory and processing stuff sometimes. Hopefully these are not permanent.

June 10, 2007: A month ago when we went for Van's Weber visit and fourth treatment, Weber told us the PET scan showed that the sarcoidosis was still active. The chest nodes were smaller but there were many active subcutaneous sites like on his arm and leg (both were biopsied and found to be granulomas). Because of this, he said he couldn't treat Van—didn't want to push the envelope and put Van in the hospital.

We were disappointed—then Weber told us that people who have such strong reactions as Van don't relapse. He followed this with a prescription to "go and live your life."

We were stunned and overcome with emotion. I don't know if he's right, but it's nice to feel we have a reprieve. I pray the melanoma is stopped. And if not for good, at least for a very long time.

We are ready for our marathon in Alaska in two weeks—maybe more than we've ever been.

June 3 we went to San Diego and cheered on our 80 teammates doing the Rock 'n' Roll Marathon. We stayed with the team at the Manchester Hyatt (next to the convention center) and went with them to the pasta party. In honor of Melanie Fastrup, I held my sign that said "THANK YOU TNT FROM A LEUKEMIA SURVIVOR." We stood at mile 6 and mile 13.1, the half marathon finish line. We saw Gail Stephens come in to the half—a big thrill! Many, many people yelled thank you to me, gave me high fives, and held thumbs up. Several wanted their photo taken with me, and several said, "I'm a survivor too." Some cried. It was a most gratifying experience.

It was during this time that we commenced the remodel of our house. Our contractor was ripping out walls, putting in drywall in our bedroom, redoing our bathroom, and building a walk-in closet. I spent most of the time holed up in the guest bedroom with fevers and chronic coughs trying to stay away from the dust. Just as I began to feel better, the carpet went in to finish the remodel, and I moved back into the bedroom and my own bed. How nice that was, and I was becoming convinced that the notion I was going to die was premature. Life was good.

My strength returned, and Virginia's tests continued to show her leukemia undetectable. We began to walk again and then to run. We began to enjoy our visits with friends. I had a biopsy of another bump on my knee and another on my neck. They were sarcoids, not melanoma. We both got stronger and stronger. We began to run more. On June 23, we flew to walk our fourth Alaska marathon. Virginia was the featured speaker at the pre-event pasta party. She is asked to do these talks because she is always inspirational, but this one was by far the best of her presentations. As I have already said, Virginia is profoundly grateful to The Leukemia & Lymphoma Society for granting support for the research that gave the world Gleevec, the drug that saved her life; and that gratitude extends to past and present walkers and runners who raise money that supports the activities of the LLS. She has gotten pretty good at expressing that gratitude in the arena of public speaking. She ended her talk by thanking the audience for helping her to find a way to remove the fear from her soul. I gave her that line, and she spoke for me too. She was also honored as one of the top national fundraisers in the nation. As always, I was proud of her, but I didn't have time to dwell on it. I had a marathon to walk the next day.

I did indeed walk my fourth Alaska Marathon. Virginia's cousin Tom kept at my side to make sure I didn't get in trouble. At about mile 20, he stopped, turned to me, and said that he was glad he didn't have to walk the marathon alone. He had thought he was going to lose me. Good friend, that Tom. It had been hard to get to the finish line, but it was so sweet to have proof that I had overcome. When I later told Virginia about my conversation with Tom, she broke down and told me that everyone thought I was going to die. I could remember times when people had thought the same about her. As with all my marathons, this one had unique local flavors. I saw a bald eagle watching over my progress and saw three moose along the route. The marathon in Alaska felt like a metaphor for my struggle against metastatic melanoma.

We ended the trip by taking a side trip to Nome, whose claim to fame is that it is the terminus of the Iditarod.

June 21-27, 2007: Alaska Marathon: I felt honored to be able to give my speech at this event. People were there from all over the country. I was very nervous about doing it right and was glad to finally get it done. It must have gone well because many, many people came up to me to tell me how inspiring it was—including John Bingham, AKA the Penguin, who was the emcee and said it was the best survivor speech he'd heard—and he'd heard plenty.

It was a kick to meet him and to know he thought I'd done a good job inspiring and thanking the crowd.

On race day, many people made a point of letting me know they appreciated my talk and said they thought of me during the race. People also came up to me at the hotel and on the streets of Anchorage to thank me and give positive comments. It was such an ego booster.

It means more to me than I can express to know I was able to relate to a national TNT audience what my experience with cancer has been and to thank them for being my partners in my fight to survive. To be successful in making that audience understand the miracle and how they contributed to it makes my heart proud. I will always remember that night—always and forever.

July—September 2007:

—My bone density scan came back normal. My doctor said I have the bones of a thirty-year-old woman!!

—My echocardiogram and stress test showed a good heart function.

—My mammogram in May showed no abnormalities.

—My July 2 PCR was negative! This makes one full year of PCR tests that read PH+ undetectable.

I am grateful for all this. Every time I go in for things like this, I worry I will have some complication that my CML/Gleevec will make even more complicated. Lots of anxiety over this. I'm so grateful when all is well. I know that if some other kind of cancer rears its head, I'll be a dead duck with my compromised platelets and red blood cells. I pray I keep safe from that.

The July 12 PET-CT scan for Van came back clear. Chest nodes are smaller. There are other small sarcoids, but Weber is not concerned.

We go to Catalina Island for my tenth anniversary of survival.

I celebrated that we'd had almost three months of respite from cancer treatment. It's been wonderful to breathe in the air peacefully.

On July 1, Virginia and I celebrated our fortieth anniversary with a party for our family and friends. It is simply impossible to describe the joy of such an event. We survived because we supported each other and were supported by others. We had excellent health care, but still, it is so hard to grasp the improbability of us both being saved from what were supposed to be fatal diseases by our separate clinical trials. But there we were, still alive and well and together. I felt pretty damned good.

I have not entirely escaped the medical profession. I still have to have PET-CT scans every three months. It is hard not to worry despite good news. I couldn't shake my skepticism. Dr. Weber has given me enough bad news that I know he was being honest about his positive projections for me. But here I thought he might simply be wrong. I had a particularly hard time telling people my good news. It might not be true, or superstitiously I thought if I brandished the news, my hubris might change something true to something not true. I asked Virginia if she felt the same way after being made healthy again. Of course she does. We don't think either of us will ever feel cancer-free, but this story is not about being cured. It is about perseverance in a battle against a powerful enemy.

It is hard to explain what it is like to get your life back. In July, we went to Bridgeport again, and it was like the first day we had been there.

We also began to participate in a flurry of races. We did a 5K in Upland, where I placed second in my age group. I did the Long Beach Half Marathon and flew compared to anything I had done before. Next came the Santa Monica 5K, where I got my personal best. After this I was first in my age group at the Calabasas 5K. I was also the only one in my age group. I was technically first and last in my age group, but the medal was gold just the same.

September 26, 2007: I've suffered mega-anxiety over the potential results of Van's scan. I can't dispel a sense of impending doom. Van has been feeling great. His "old self" is back, and he's been writing about our experiences these past ten years. My journal and documentation of our medical experiences for Van have helped jog memories. I pray this day's scans will be in the happy category, but my mind dwells on the possibilities—will something else show up? If so, what will we do? Dr. Weber will not be at Norris after next Friday. He will be at Moffitt Cancer Center in Florida. Where will Van be going for treatment after this? How very long and hard the medical appointment trips will be! My soul and heart pray the melanoma has been stopped, but I can't help feeling unsettled—without a plan. Both Van and I know he needs someone local, but he is putting off connecting with O'Day.

The fear this disease puts in one's soul is sometimes paralyzing. And after years of dealing with each challenge it has placed in your path, you begin to realize what a roller coaster ride you're on. Nothing is certain; anything can happen; there is no safe haven. You just have to rely on yourself to weather the storm and realize you can't depend on calm waters staying with you for very long.

October 5, 2007: The scans came back clear! Weber suggested that Van stay with Norris but follow up with him in January in Florida, at Moffitt. We decided to do that.

My September PCR came back undetectable. Yea!

I am grateful for a respite from cancer worries for the two of us. Every cell in my body hopes this lasts for a long time.

In November, Tom, Virginia and I did the Santa Barbara Half Marathon for the fifth time. To make up for the one I was forced to skip, I had the best time of my life. We felt so good, both mentally and physically. As Tom says, when you are in trouble, you have to put your head down into the wind and move forward. We did that, and we did it together. It is impossible after something like this to go back to your old life. You might be holding onto pieces of what was the past, but now it has a different context. A wonderful context all the same.

On December 6, 2007, Virginia and I flew to Atlanta for the 2007 ASH meeting, which was the seventh for me and the fourth for her. We learned that in a follow-up study of a group of early patients on Gleevec, an amazing 93 percent had survived. Brilliant researchers dig in deeper to ensure these numbers remain high or higher. Dasatinib had finished trials with great results, had been approved by the FDA, and was already salvaging some very sick people. Another drug, a Novartis second-generation drug called nilotinib, had also been approved and was saving patients as well. And many more drugs to help CML patients were in the pipeline. The new drugs did have side effects that had not been anticipated. Dasatinib, in particular, had a greater effect on platelet production, so some patients were having seriously low platelet counts. With Virginia's platelet problems, if we had jumped at a chance to change to dasatinib, it might have been a disaster.

It was also becoming clear that a portion of the patients who were resistant to treatment had no mutations. A number of papers summarized research that showed some patients simply could not absorb their drugs as well as others and therefore had levels in their blood that were below a therapeutic level.

We were able to see Dr. Sawyers and Dr. Shah again. Dr. Shah told Virginia that she was going to be fine. This time we believed him. These two researchers' investigations are expanding into other cancers; they are destined to life-saving accomplishments.

The number of CML survivors when Virginia was first diagnosed had been around 35,000. By 2007 this number was 100,000, and that is expected to level out at 250,000. There was some discussion at ASH about the profits accrued by the pharmaceutical companies that develop and produce drugs for CML patients. Yearly patient costs for these drugs average $50,000, so the potential for revenue is clear. It is little wonder that other companies are scrambling to get a piece of the action. We remain eternally grateful to Novartis for Gleevec, but controversy remains about the financial burdens put on people whose primary goal in life is to survive—about the financial barriers to life-saving treatment.

Still, we visited the huge Novartis booth at the conference, and Virginia was recognized by many of the sales reps who had been at the Century City meeting. They and we know that something special has happened and no matter the price, a great many people are alive today because of what has been accomplished.

On December 17, I had another PET/CT scan in preparation for my January meeting in Florida with Dr. Weber. My anxiety level rose, and I searched my body obsessively for lumps and bumps. I guess I will never stop wondering if and when this disease will come back.

December 17, 2007: Once again I sit waiting while Van is having his three-month follow-up PET-CT scan at USC PET Imaging. This time we will get a CD and have the results faxed to Dr. Weber in Tampa, Florida. We go there on January 16.

As the days led up to today, my anxiety level rose higher and higher. What will this scan show? What happens if there are problems? Do we go to Angeles Clinic and Dr. O'Day? Do we see Weber anyway? Our flights are already booked.

Van's hip has been hurting—the one that had the surgery. Of course, right away you wonder if the tumor has returned. Or could it be the scar tissue? Van has complained of being tired the past couple or three weeks. Is the cancer back? Or is he just tired? Is he also anxious or depressed about possible outcomes of this test today and feeling tired because of that? I know he's under stress because he has been a bit abrupt several times lately—very uncharacteristic of his usually even personality.

Here's the thing—we have absolutely no control over this, and that drives me over the edge. You just sit tight and wait until you learn your fate.

I am so grateful for these past three months of freedom from illness and worry. I hope it's not asking too much to have three more. I can't help but register in my consciousness that it was exactly a year ago that scans showed the enlarged nodes in Van's chest and two years ago that they showed the tumors in the hip and jejunum. This month is a bad one for scans, it seems. I hope we can break the mold today. I am filled with foreboding—experience teaches me to have these feelings. I'm wearing my little guardian angel dog that I wear to all Van's and my medical appointments. Someone gave me this dog—maybe Judy—when I was going to UCLA for the trial, and I began wearing it then. It's gotten us through so much over these past years. I can only hope it continues to be on guard for us.

The PET nurse just told me they can give us the CD but not the written report until we see a physician.

So there you are. We'll be in the dark until we see him in Florida. It's a big pain in the neck.

During the period between Christmas and New Year's, I have historically gone through my old research papers to see what is important and what I can discard as outdated. Doing this, I ran into a 2003 research paper out of Berkeley on ipilimumab. I hadn't remembered that studies on this inhibitor had been going on that long, but I had quite a little record of articles to prove it. At the end of the paper, the author thanked all his supporters and lo and behold, he thanked The Leukemia & Lymphoma Society. Once again I found a demonstration that cancer research, no matter how focused, no matter what disease it addresses, is likely to have implications for other cancers as well. The article is a reminder that organizations like the LLS are the ones that support early research that can't yet garner the big government grants. And so the LLS played an important role in saving both Virginia and me.

During this time, Virginia read some of what I had written. Referring to this period, she once asked, "Did you ever wonder what was going on in my mind during this time?" I had no answer. She then shared her journals, and we weaved our story together into the book you're reading.

On January 3, I received an e-mail from Dr. Weber to let me know that the reports on my scans had arrived in his office and they looked good. We began investigating tourist spots in Florida that we might visit. We were spiritually and physically feeling very good.

Ending this story has been a challenge. After ten years of fighting, our battle with cancer came to an abrupt and nearly unbelievable end. The abruptness was akin to the end of any endurance event we have run or walked, where a seemingly never-ending experience in fact ends the instant the finish line is crossed.

And so we have had a difficult time ending our story. In fact, I wrote a chapter that continued to describe our lives. I described marathon after marathon, half marathon after half marathon. I mentioned the perfect scans and tests and congratulated Virginia for all the new awards she received from The Leukemia & Lymphoma Society. She was even recognized by one of her alma maters as the Distinguished Alumnae of the Year for Community Service. I went into detail about how I triumphantly finished the 2008 L.A. Marathon, erasing the disaster of 2007. I then went on to talk about how we continued to worry, but that we were no longer terrorized by our cancers. We had chased our miracles, and we had adjusted to our victory.

We thought we were immune from constant cancer concerns, until I received a report on a recent biopsy taken by my dermatologist and I realized that with cancer, there is always another race—and another finish line to conquer.

DIAGNOSIS:

UPPER BACK, 4 MM PUNCH:

DISPLASTIC COMPOUND NEVUS WITH SEVER ARCHTECTURE DISORDER AND CYTOLOGIC ATYPIA, SUSPICIOUS FOR MALIGNANT MELANOMA, EXTENDING TO ONE OF TWO LATERAL BIOPSY MARGINS (SEE COMMENT).

COMMENT:

Additional three levels on specimen A are examined, which supports the above diagnosis. Recommend complete excision of the lesion with margin.

Virginia and I decided we would always fear the return of cancer. We would more than worry. We would always fear, and that was probably for the best. I am still grateful for every day. And Virginia does her best to focus on the day she is in.

October 6, 2008: When I signed up for the L.A. Marathon with

Team in Training, it never occurred to me that I would become an expert in marathoning. Now, nine years, two full marathons, and twenty or so half marathons later, I hope I am close to the finish line of the marathon of our lives—standing up to cancer. When I think back on the past decade, I don't know how I got through it all. I'm sure the odds of both Van and me being diagnosed with terminal cancers are fairly low, but I know the odds of us both being saved by science and brilliant physician researchers are even lower. We are living a miracle.

Still, I can't in my heart feel like I'm looking at the finish line. My cancer experience has taught me that nothing is as it may seem. I still go from one PCR undetectable test to the other waiting for the other shoe to drop, even while having the feeling that maybe I'm going to remain this way for a long time. Both Van and I still sink into anxiety and fear when he has to go for his follow-up scans and we still endure the hellish waiting for the results. Every bump or lump on Van's body, every pain, and every ache sends me back for a little clip of the despair I felt just a few months ago. I can't look into the future. I've learned not to. I just take each day for what it is to me—a joy to experience while healthy and well.

It's become clear to me that my marathon training has taught me more than how to walk/run 26.2 or 13.1 miles and cross the finish line. I've been involved in the marathon of my life these past eleven years, especially the last seven with Van's standing up to the monster melanoma. There have been times I was so weary, I wanted to curl up on the sidelines and shut out the world. There have been times when I was so angry, I wanted to blow up the world. There have been times when I was in such despair, I felt we weren't going to make it. But I kept on. I didn't know any other way. I just gritted my teeth and kept putting one foot in front of the other, and here I am: still strong, still standing up, armed with a new awareness and perception of what it is to live.

I can only say that I wake up every day and give thanks for our health and for each other. Is the finish line in sight? I don't know, and I'm not willing to say. I only know that today at least, life is good.

I don't know how the biopsy of the complete excision will turn out, but it has already served to remind us that we will never be free of cancer—though we are grateful for the days we have had in defiance of the odds. Recently we read news that Dr. Brian Druker was granted $100,000,000 for more cancer research from one of the founders of Nike. We saw Barack Obama elected president, and I get to see my sweet wife's face every morning. But the fact is that these wonderful facts of life only whet our appetites for more days than we have had, and we will continue to fight and chase our miracles.

As corny as it all seems, Virginia and I have never done anything to threaten the love and devotion we have for each other. We know we aren't the only couple deeply bonded, but we are certainly one of them. This is why Virginia's cancer is my cancer and mine is also hers. I think it is fair to say that we have been through a lot, learned a lot, and survived the most improbable set of circumstances because we fought tooth and nail to save each other. It's a victory that has bought us sweet time. But that doesn't mean things last forever. They don't. But we continue to squeeze every day of joy out of our lives together and we intend to keep this love story going as long as our spirits allow.

Epilogue

The book *Journey to the Finish Line* ends in the last months of 2008 with the improbable survival of us both. We are still alive and active in 2017. Although we both have been through some scares since, they all turned out to be diagnostic mistakes. Both of us are still running as an affirmation of our healthy lives and as a way to raise funds for cancer research. Together we have completed more than two hundred marathons and half marathons and have raised over half a million dollars, and we will do this until we can't.

Our care providers have been awarded commensurate with the level of their incredible accomplishment. Douglas Blaney went on to be president of the American Society of Clinical Oncology and Medical Director of Stanford Cancer Center where he is now a Professor of Medicine. Jeffrey Weber is now Deputy Director of the Perlmutter Cancer Center of NYU Langone. He runs a research team and is a prolific publisher of articles, especially involving immunotherapy. We travel to see him because he is still Van's doctor. Brian Druker is now the Director of the Knight Cancer Center at Oregon Health and Science University in Portland, Oregon. Charles Sawyers is now Chair of the Human Oncology and Pathogenesis Program at Memorial Sloan Kettering in New York City. James Allison is now Executive Director of Immunotherapy at M.D. Anderson Cancer Center at the University of Texas, Houston. Brian Druker, Charles Sawyers, and James Allison have received many awards for their work. Each has received the United States' most prestigious award for their work, the Lasker-De Bakey Clinical Medical Research Award. This places all three within spitting distance from a Nobel Prize.

We understand now that we were in seminal clinical trials that were the culmination of a process where groups of talented people, working together, advanced not just our understanding of cancer, but also the way we treat it. Specifically, tyrosine kinase inhibitors like Gleevec that target individual cancer cells became both a treatment for specific cancers, and representatives of a paradigm shift that opened a new field of research and treatment with tremendous potential. Checkpoint inhibitors like ipilimumab, now known as Yervoy, saved melanoma patients who would have otherwise died, while they also open the door to research that is showing that an individual's immune system can be manipulated to see and eradicate many other cancers. The insights derived from our trials will be built upon. We also know there are new groups of people out there, who we do not know, whose backs are to the wall who are preparing to enter clinical trials. We hope that these desperate, but brave people are going to get what we got, lives full and free of fear. And if we are at all lucky, they will advance knowledge and thus treatment and cures in the war on cancer. The end is when cancer is totally eradicated, when the war on cancer is over. Our experiences give us a profound belief that the human talent is there to make this happen. So our end is not the end. It is the beginning. The beginning of the road to a cure.

Authors' Note

Thank you for joining us in our story of fighting and surviving cancer. If you loved the book and have a few moments, we would really appreciate a short review on the page or site where you bought the book. Reviews from readers like you make a huge difference in helping new readers find our story, and we greatly appreciate your help in spreading the word.

Thank you!

Virginia and Van Garner

www.ingramcontent.com/pod-product-compliance
Lightning Source LLC
Chambersburg PA
CBHW060040030426

42334CB00019B/2416